The Official
Rails-to-Trails
Conservancy
Guidebook

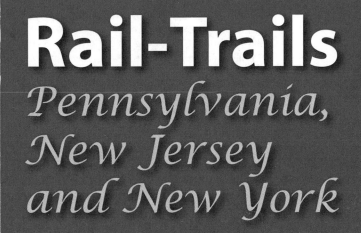

Rail-Trails

*Pennsylvania,
New Jersey
and New York*

D0107463

Rail-Trails Pennsylvania, New Jersey and New York

1st EDITION 2011
3rd printing 2011

Copyright © 2011 by Rails-to-Trails Conservancy

Front cover photographs copyright © 2011 by Rails-to-Trails Conservancy
Interior photographs are by Rails-to-Trails Conservancy, except for the following
contributed by others, with our special thanks: Photos on pages 7, 11, 13, 19, 27,
29, 35 (top), 36, 39, 57 (top), 63, 71 (top), 72, 75, 85, 103 (top), 104, 107, 119, 125,
126, 129, 130, 135 (top), 141, 151, 269, and 311 from Boyd Loving; page 35, Teresa
Rose; page 163, Valley Wellness Trails Partnership, Active Living by Design;
page 281, Dee Columbus; page 297, Debra Frawley, Council on Greenways and
Trails; and page 345, Malcolm Sias.
Maps: Tim Rosner and Lohnes+Wright
Cover design: Lisa Pletka and Scott McGrew
Interior design and layout: Lisa Pletka and Larry B. Van Dyke
Editors: Jennifer Kaleba and Karen Stewart

ISBN 978-0-89997-649-5

Manufactured in the United States of America

Published by: **Wilderness Press**
Keen Communications
PO Box 43673
Birmingham, AL 35243
(800) 443-7227; fax (205) 326-1012
info@wildernesspress.com
www.wildernesspress.com

Visit our website for a complete listing of our books and for ordering information.

Distributed by Publishers Group West

Cover photos: North County Trailway *(main)*; Lehigh Gorge State Park Trail *(inset top)*; Paulinskill Valley Trail *(inset bottom)*; and Lycoming Creek Bikeway *(back cover)*
Frontispiece: John Bartram Trail, a segment of the Schuylkill River Trail

About Rails-to-Trails Conservancy

Headquartered in Washington, D.C., Rails-to-Trails Conservancy (RTC) fosters one great mission: to protect America's irreplaceable rail corridors by transforming them into multiuse trails. Its hope is that these pathways will reconnect Americans with their neighbors, communities, nature and proud history.

Railways helped build America. Spanning from coast to coast, these ribbons of steel linked people, communities, and enterprises, spurring commerce and forging a single nation that bridges a continent. But in recent decades, many of these routes have fallen into disuse, severing communal ties that helped bind Americans together.

When RTC opened its doors in 1986, the rail-trail movement was in its infancy. While there were some 250 miles of open rail-trails in the United States, most projects focused on single, linear routes in rural areas, created for recreation and conservation. RTC sought broader protection for the unused corridors, incorporating rural, suburban and urban routes.

Year after year, RTC's efforts to protect and align public funding with trail building created an environment that allowed trail advocates in communities all across the country to initiate trail projects. These ever-growing ranks of trail professionals, volunteers and RTC supporters have built momentum for the national rail-trails movement. As the number of supporters multiplied, so too did the rail-trails. By the turn of the 21st century, there were some 1,100 rail-trails on the ground, and RTC recorded nearly 84,000 supporters, from business leaders and politicians to environmentalists and healthy-living advocates.

Americans now enjoy more than 19,000 miles of open rail-trails. And as they flock to the trails to commune with neighbors, neighborhoods and nature, their economic, physical and environmental wellness continue to flourish.

In 2011, Rails-to-Trails Conservancy celebrated 25 years of creating, protecting, serving and connecting rail-trails. Boasting more than 150,000 members and supporters, RTC is the nation's leading advocate for trails and greenways.

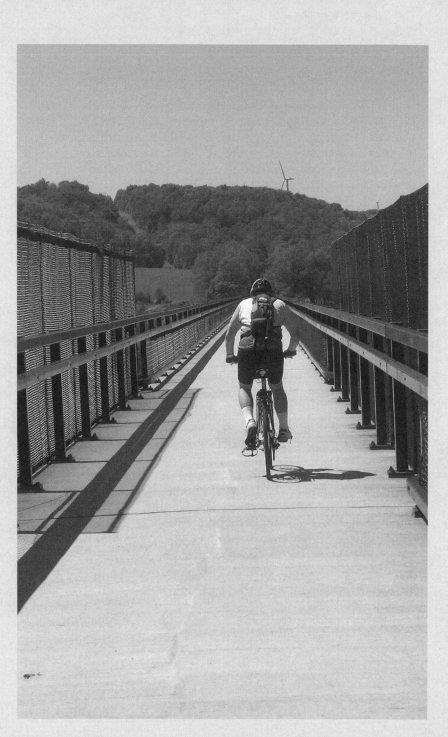

Running from Pittsburgh, Pennsylvania, to Cumberland, Maryland, the Great Allegheny Passage traces the paths of railroads that helped build America.

Foreword

Dear Reader:

For those of you who have already experienced the sheer enjoyment and freedom of riding on a rail-trail, welcome back! You'll find *Rail-Trails Pennsylvania, New Jersey and New York* to be a useful and fun guide to your favorite trails, as well as an introduction to pathways you have yet to travel.

For readers who are discovering, for the first time, the adventures you can have on a rail-trail, thank you for joining the rail-trail movement. Since 1986, Rails-to-Trails Conservancy has been the No. 1 supporter and defender of these priceless public corridors. We are excited to bring you *Rail-Trails Pennsylvania, New Jersey and New York* so you, too, can enjoy this region's rail-trails.

Built on unused, former railroad corridors, these hiking and biking trails are an ideal way to connect with your community, with nature, and with your friends and family. I've found that rail-trails have a way of bringing people together, and as you'll see from this book, there are opportunities in every state you visit to get on a trail. Whether you're looking for a place to exercise, explore, commute, or play—there is a rail-trail in this book for you.

So I invite you to sit back, relax, pick a trail that piques your interest—and then get out, get active, and have some fun. I'll be out on the trails, too, so be sure to wave as you go by.

Happy Trails,

Keith Laughlin
President, Rails-to-Trails Conservancy

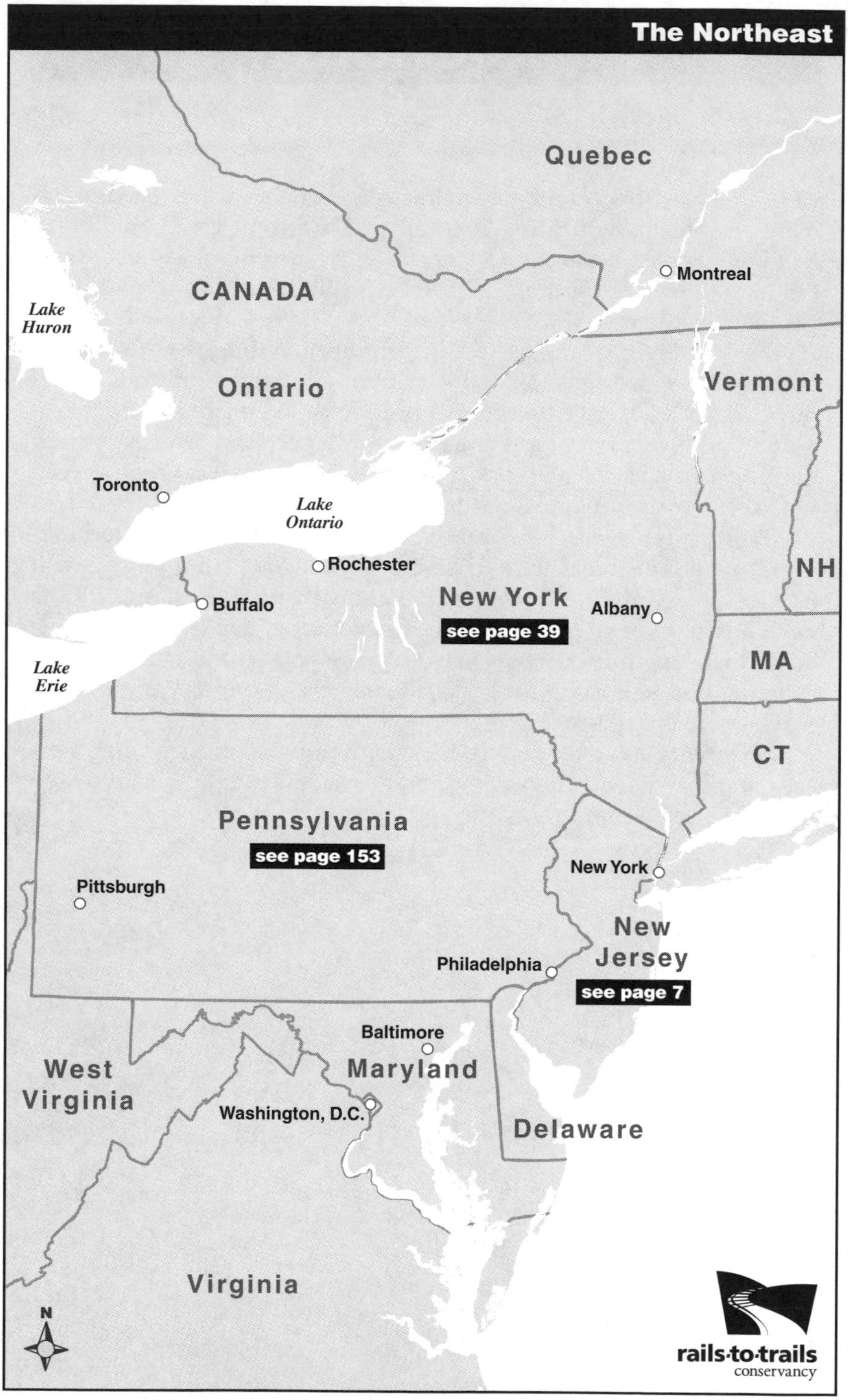

Quebec

CANADA

Lake
Huron

○ Montreal

Ontario

Vermont

Toronto ○

Lake
Ontario

○ Rochester

New York

NH

Albany ○

○ Buffalo

see page 39

Lake
Erie

MA

CT

Pennsylvania

see page 153

New York ○

Pittsburgh
○

New
Jersey

Philadelphia ○

see page 7

Baltimore
○

West
Virginia

Maryland

Washington, D.C. ○

Delaware

Virginia

N

rails·to·trails
conservancy

Contents

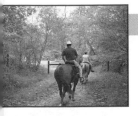

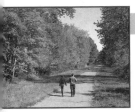

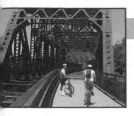

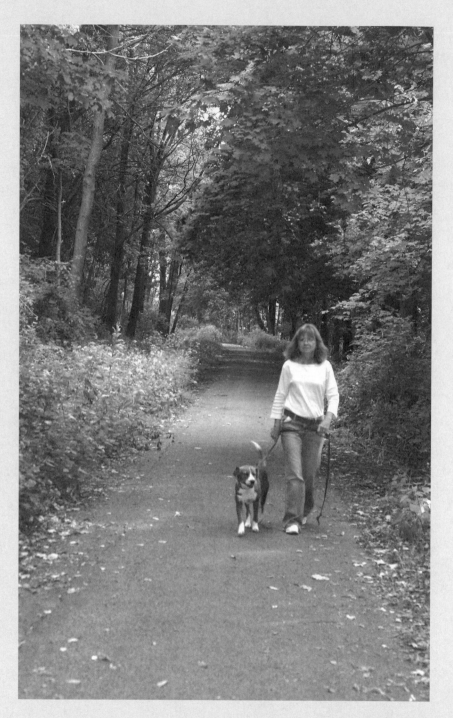

If you are traveling in the area east of the Hudson River and want to stretch your legs, the Uncle Sam Bike Trail offers a scenic retreat.

INTRODUCTION

Every which way you turn in the Northeast, you're bound to find a rail-trail. The region has one of the highest concentrations of rail-trails in the country, stemming largely from the area's dense population centers, industrial heritage, port cities and canalways. Simply put, a lot of trains once moved a lot of people and goods through this part of the country—and often still do. *Rail-Trails Pennsylvania, New Jersey and New York* covers the rail-trails, rail-with-trails and even several towpaths of Pennsylvania, New Jersey and New York. Of the more than 1,600 rail-trails in the country, we've selected 105 diverse rail-trails in the Northeast to share in *Rail-Trails Pennsylvania, New Jersey and New York*, each one serving as a window into the world the railroad once served.

Visit New Jersey's Columbia Trail, an 11.3-mile pathway that wends through the magnificent Ken Lockwood Gorge where steep slopes reveal rapid water and dramatic rock formations. A naturalist's dream, the surrounding hardwood forest makes for a particularly colorful autumn, and in spring wildflowers brighten the landscape.

Everything old is new again on New York's High Line, a raised corridor that spans nearly a mile of the lower Manhattan skyway, preserving the old railroad line as a walking trail and garden oasis for millions of New York City dwellers. Or journey beyond the city to the Walkway Over the Hudson, a renovated steel-truss bridge stretching approximately 1.25 miles across and 212 feet above the Hudson River.

In Pennsylvania—a state that clocks in with 146 rail-trails, the most rail-trails of all 50 states—you're spoiled for choice. Take a multi-day journey on the 152-mile Great Allegheny Passage, or enjoy a speedy out-and-back on the 4-mile Greater Hazleton Rails to Trails. Get your dose of history as you travel 20.5 miles from Philadelphia to Valley Forge on the Schuylkill River Trail, or cross the state line into Ohio on the 10-mile Stavich Bicycle Trail.

No matter which route in *Rail-Trails Pennsylvania, New Jersey and New York* you decide to try, you'll be touching on the heart of the community that helped build it and the history that first brought the rails to the region.

What is a Rail-Trail?

Rail-trails are multiuse public paths built along former railroad corridors. Most often flat or following a gentle grade, they are suited to walking, running, cycling, mountain biking, inline skating, cross-country skiing, horseback riding and wheelchair use. Since the 1960s, Americans have created more than 19,000 miles of rail-trails throughout the country.

These extremely popular recreation and transportation corridors traverse urban, suburban and rural landscapes. Many preserve historic landmarks, while others serve as wildlife conservation corridors, linking isolated parks and establishing greenways in developed areas. Rail-trails also stimulate local economies by boosting tourism and promoting trailside businesses.

What is a Rail-with-Trail?

A rail-with-trail is a public path that parallels a still-active rail line. Some run adjacent to high-speed, scheduled trains, often linking public transportation stations, while others follow tourist routes and slow-moving excursion trains. Many share an easement, separated from the rails by extensive fencing. There are more than 115 rails-with-trails in the U.S.

HOW TO USE THIS BOOK

*R*ail-Trails *Pennsylvania, New Jersey and New York* provides the information you need to plan a rewarding rail-trail trek. With words to inspire you and maps to chart your path, it makes choosing the best route a breeze. Following are some of the highlights.

Maps

You'll find three levels of maps in this book: an overall regional map, state locator maps, and detailed trail maps.

The northeastern region includes New Jersey, New York and Pennsylvania. Each chapter details a particular state's network of trails, marked on locator maps in the chapter introduction. Use these maps to find the trails nearest you, or select several neighboring trails and plan a weekend hiking or biking excursion. Once you find a trail on a state locator map, simply flip to the corresponding page number for a full description. Accompanying trail maps mark each route's access roads, trailheads, parking areas, restrooms and other defining features.

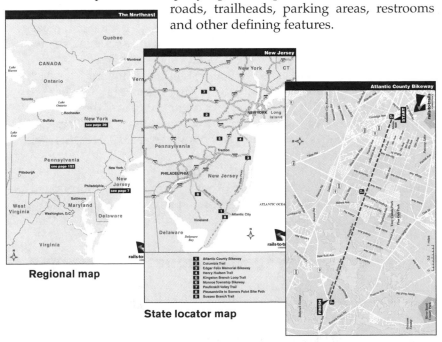

Regional map

State locator map

Trail map

Trail Descriptions

Trails are listed in alphabetical order within each chapter. Each description leads off with a set of summary information, including trail endpoints and mileage, a roughness index, the trail surface, and possible uses.

The map and summary information list the trail endpoints (either a city, street, or more specific location), with suggested points from which to start and finish. Additional access points are marked on the maps and mentioned in the trail descriptions. The maps and descriptions also highlight available amenities, including parking and restrooms, as well as such area attractions as shops, services, museums, parks and stadiums. Trail length is listed in miles.

Each trail bears a roughness index rating from 1 to 3. A rating of 1 indicates a smooth, level surface that is accessible to users of all ages and abilities. A 2 rating means the surface may be loose and/or uneven and could pose a problem for road bikes and wheelchairs. A 3 rating suggests a rough surface that is only recommended for mountain bikers and hikers. Surfaces can range from asphalt or concrete to ballast, cinder, crushed stone, gravel, grass, dirt and/or sand. Where relevant, trail descriptions address alternating surface conditions.

All rail-trails are open to pedestrians, and most allow bicycles, except where noted in the trail summary or description. The summary also indicates wheelchair access. Other possible uses include inline skating, mountain biking, hiking, horseback riding, fishing and cross-country skiing. While most trails are off-limits to motor vehicles, some local trail organizations do allow ATVs and snowmobiles.

Trail descriptions themselves suggest an ideal itinerary for each route, including the best parking areas and access points, where to begin, your direction of travel, and any highlights along the way. The text notes any connecting or neighboring routes, with page numbers for the respective trail descriptions. Following each description are directions to the recommended trailheads.

Each trail description also lists a local contact (name, address, phone number, and website) for further information. Be sure to call these trail managers or volunteer groups in advance for updates and current conditions.

Key to Map Icons

Parking

Drinking water

Bathrooms

Trail Use

Rail-trails are popular routes for a range of uses, often making them busy places to play. Trail etiquette applies. If passing other trail users on your bicycle, always try to pass on the left with an audible warning such as a bike-mounted bell or a polite but firm, "Passing on your left!" For your safety and that of other trail users, keep children and pets from straying into oncoming trail traffic. Keep dogs leashed, and supervise children until they can demonstrate proper behavior.

Cyclists and inline skaters should wear helmets, reflective clothing, and other safety gear, as some trails involve hazardous road crossings. It's also best to bring a flashlight or bike- or helmet-mounted light for tunnel passages or twilight excursions.

Key to Trail Use

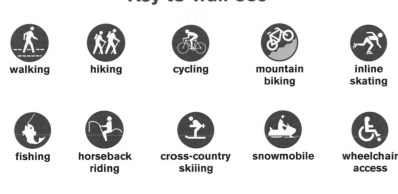

| walking | hiking | cycling | mountain biking | inline skating |
| fishing | horseback riding | cross-country skiiing | snowmobile | wheelchair access |

Learn More

While *Rail-Trails Pennsylvania, New Jersey and New York* is a helpful guide to available routes in the region, it wasn't feasible to list every rail-trail in these three states, and new rail-trails spring up each year. To learn about additional rail-trails in your area or to plan a trip to an area beyond the scope of this book, log on to the Rails-to-Trails Conservancy home page (www.railstotrails.org) and click on the Find a Trail link. RTC's online database lists more than 1,600 rail-trails nationwide, searchable by state, county, city, trail name, surface type, length, activity and/or keywords regarding your interest. A number of listings include photos and reviews from people who've already visited the trail.

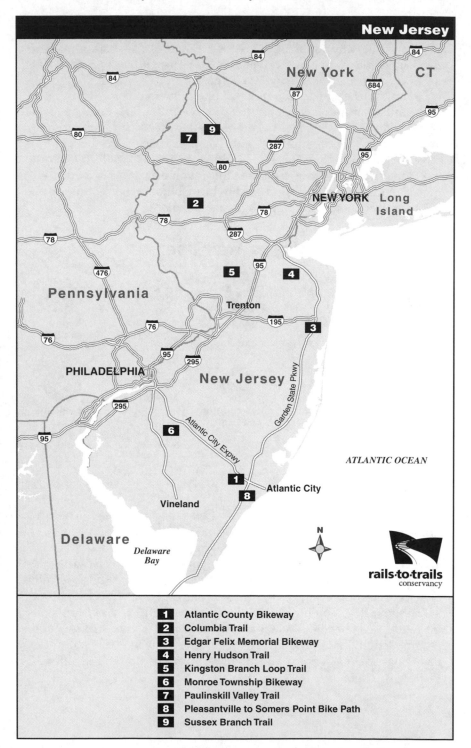

New Jersey

New York   CT

NEW YORK   Long Island

Pennsylvania

Trenton

PHILADELPHIA

New Jersey

Atlantic City

Vineland

ATLANTIC OCEAN

Delaware

Delaware Bay

N

rails·to·trails
conservancy

1	Atlantic County Bikeway
2	Columbia Trail
3	Edgar Felix Memorial Bikeway
4	Henry Hudson Trail
5	Kingston Branch Loop Trail
6	Monroe Township Bikeway
7	Paulinskill Valley Trail
8	Pleasantville to Somers Point Bike Path
9	Sussex Branch Trail

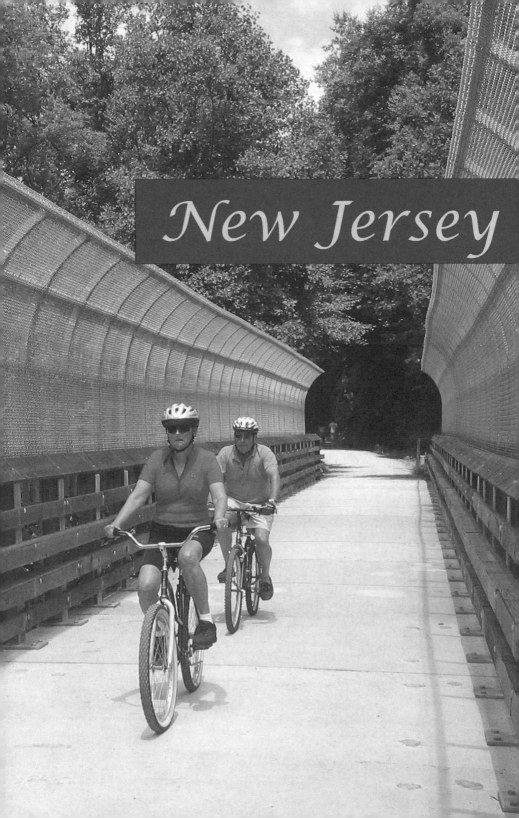

New Jersey

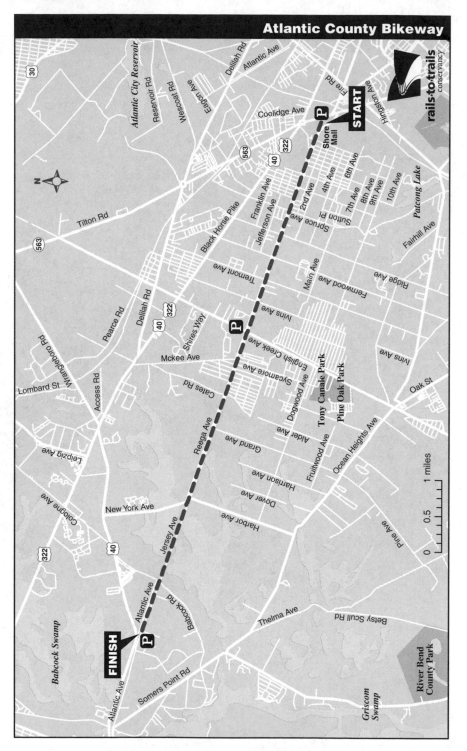

Atlantic County Bikeway

The 7.5-mile Atlantic County Bikeway offers a relaxing escape from the crush of traffic surrounding Atlantic City, the beachfront gaming and resort town. The trail is situated 9 miles west of Atlantic City, near the nexus of the heavily traveled Atlantic City Expressway and the Garden State Parkway. Quieter two-lane roads paralleling each end of the bikeway provide convenient trail access.

Wide swaths of mowed grass flank the clean, well-designed trail. Strategically planted trees provide a welcome buffer from the roads, and the 15 secondary road crossings are clearly marked for trail users and motorists. The trail periodically curves around utility poles, incorporating overhead electric lines into the design.

Starting at the Shore Mall the trail passes through a corridor of trees. About a half mile from the start the trail runs between Reega Avenue to the north and West Jersey Avenue to the south. The adjoining landscape is a mixture of residential neighborhoods and undeveloped woodlands.

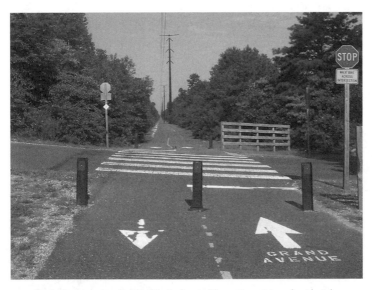

The landscape surrounding the Atlantic County Bikeway is a mixture of residential neighborhoods and undeveloped woodlands.

Location
Atlantic County

Endpoints
Shore Mall to English Creek Avenue in Mays Landing

Mileage
7.5

Roughness Index
1

Surface
Asphalt

9

A few benches make great rest spots, but places to stock up on supplies are scarce. Be sure to bring your own food and water.

DIRECTIONS

The eastern trailhead is at the north side of the Shore Mall parking lot. From Atlantic City follow State Route 322/40 (Black Horse Pike) west toward the Garden State Parkway. Cross under the parkway and turn left into the Shore Mall. Turn right and follow the outside lane of the parking lot to the north side and look for designated Atlantic County Bikeway parking.

The western section of the trail lies between the east- and west-running sides of Atlantic Avenue. The trailhead is between Atlantic Avenue and at the intersection of 19th Street. Follow Atlantic Avenue west to reach the trailhead. Parking is available on the south side of the 19th and Atlantic intersection.

There is additional parking just east of Mays Landing at the intersection of Atlantic Avenue and English Creek Avenue.

Contact: Atlantic County Parks & Recreation
109 State Highway 50
Mays Landing, NJ 08330
(609) 625-1897
www.aclink.org/PARKS

The Columbia Trail strings together forests, farms and parklands as it stretches 11 miles among the small towns of High Bridge, Califon and Long Valley. Most of the corridor parallels the South Branch of the Raritan River. After passenger trains and rail cars laden with iron ore ceased running this line, the Columbia Gas company constructed a pipeline under the former rail bed. It then transferred the surface rights to the parks departments of Hunterdon and Morris counties for a recreational trail.

The trail starts in High Bridge near the center of town. Several lightly traveled side streets intersect the corridor before you encounter woodlands and the banks of the Raritan River, considered one of the state's premier fly-fishing trout streams. In approximately a quarter mile from the starting point the Taylor Steelworkers' Historical Greenway, a 6.25-mile hiking trail through historic sites, intersects the Columbia Trail on the right.

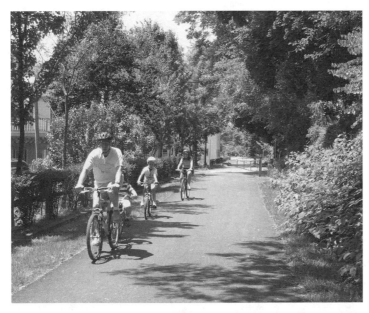

The hardwood forest of the Columbia Trail is particularly colorful.

Location
Hunterdon and Morris counties

Endpoints
Main Street in High Bridge to Schooleys Mountain Road in Long Valley

Mileage
11.3

Roughness Index
2

Surface
Crushed stone

11

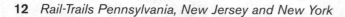

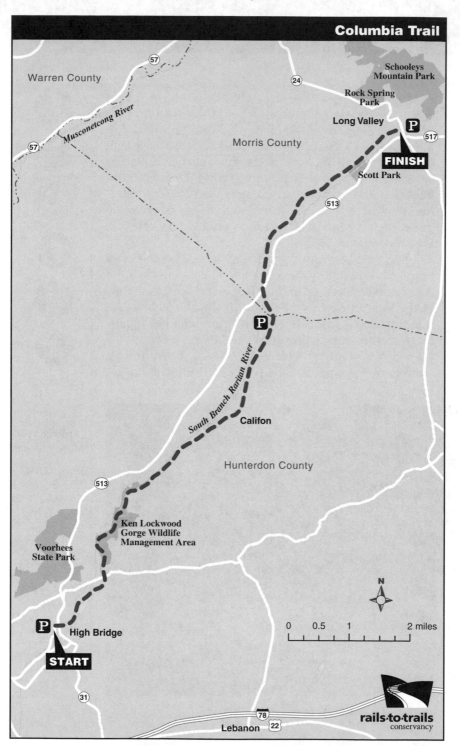

Columbia Trail

Warren County

57

Musconetcong River

57

24

Schooleys
Mountain Park

Rock Spring
Park

Long Valley

P

517

FINISH

Morris County

Scott Park

513

P

South Branch Raritan River

Califon

Hunterdon County

513

Ken Lockwood
Gorge Wildlife
Management Area

Voorhees
State Park

P

High Bridge

START

31

N

0   0.5   1   2 miles

78

Lebanon   22

rails·to·trails
conservancy

After about 2 miles, the trail enters the magnificent Ken Lockwood Gorge where steep slopes reveal rapid water and dramatic rock formations. A naturalist's dream, the gorge is named for the late outdoor writer and conservationist. The surrounding hardwood forest makes for a particularly colorful autumn, and in spring wildflowers brighten the landscape. Black bears have been spotted in the area, though far less frequently than white-tailed deer, raccoons, coyote, fox, squirrels and chipmunks.

The tiny borough of Califon boasts 170 structures on the National Register of Historic Places, including the restored railroad station. The station, built entirely of stone, houses the Califon Historical Society. The area mills gained prominence for furnishing central New Jersey's thriving agricultural industry with wooden slat baskets commonly known as peach baskets. Homes in the Victorian village are marked with the date of construction and the names of the builder rather than street addresses. Local legend says the name *Califon* was a sign painter's invention. The town was originally called California but when the railroad station was built, the sign painter could not fit the name *California* on the board provided and abbreviated it to *Califon*.

At West Valley Brook Road, the trail leaves Hunterdon County and enters Morris County. Very little, other than a change in the design of the trail access gates, changes though. The landscape along this section into the Long Valley is more agricultural in nature. Currently

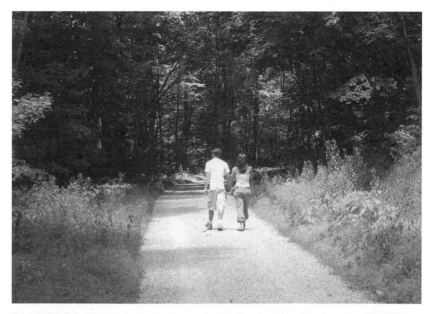

The Columbia Trail strings together forests, farms and parklands as it stretches 11 miles among the small towns of High Bridge, Califon and Long Valley.

the trail ends at Schooleys Mountain Road in Long Valley. Morris County Park Commission is awaiting easements to connect another 2 miles of trail.

DIRECTIONS

To reach the west, or High Bridge, end of the trail from Interstate 78, take the exit for State Route 31 North. Turn right on West Main Street. After crossing under the railroad tracks, turn left. Trailhead parking is on the left just past the borough hall.

To reach the east, or Long Valley, end of the trail, from Interstate 287, take the exit for US Routes 206/202 North. Bear left to remain on US Route 206. Turn left onto State Route 24. Follow Route 24 by turning right onto Schooleys Mountain Road. The trailhead parking lot is on your left.

Contact: Hunterdon County Department of Parks and Recreation
P.O. Box 2900
Flemington, NJ 08822
(908) 806-1158
www.hunterdon.nj.us/depts/parks/guides/Columbia
   Trail.htm

Morris County Park Commission
P.O. Box 1295
Morristown, NJ 07962
(973) 326-7600
www.morrisparks.net/aspparks/columbiamain.asp

Edgar Felix Memorial Bikeway

The Edgar Felix Memorial Bikeway packs enough history, scenery and activity in its 5.2 miles for an all-day adventure. Manasquan cyclist Edgar Felix lobbied his town to acquire a portion of the inactive Freehold and Jamesburg Agricultural Railroad for a trail. The first 2 miles of the bikeway opened in 1971, and in 2006 the trail became the first dedicated segment of the 55-mile Capital to Coast multi-use trail that will span New Jersey from Trenton to the beach community of Manasquan.

Heading west from Manasquan—a mere 2 miles from the Atlantic coast—the trail passes residential neighborhoods before arriving at Orchard Park recreation complex. There is limited parking for trail users adjacent to the park.

After crossing State Route 35, the trail is flanked by less densely populated residential areas and commercial enterprises. A 2-mile connecting trail on the north

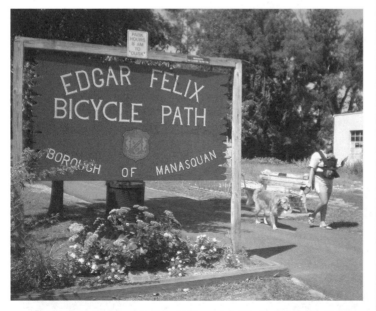

The entrance to the Edgar Felix Memorial Bikeway is just 2 miles from the Atlantic Ocean.

Location
Monmouth County

Endpoints
North Main Street in Manasquan to Allaire State Park

Mileage
5.2

Roughness Index
1

Surface
Asphalt

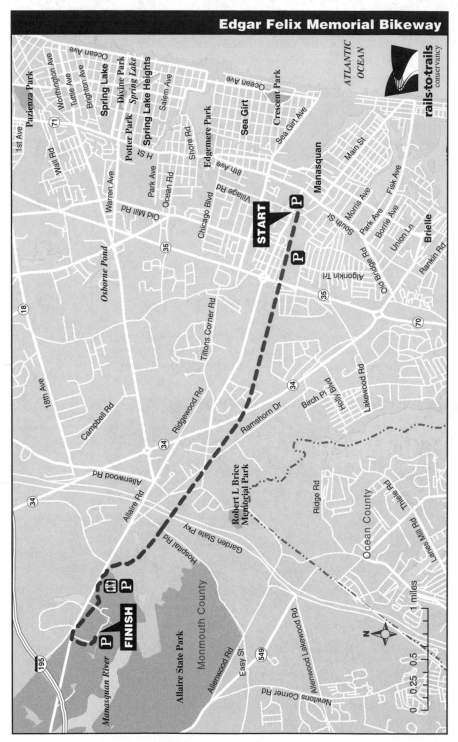

side of the bikeway provides a rolling, winding side trip to the Wall Township Municipal Complex.

After passing under State Route 34, the trail surroundings become more rural, with deeper forests and open fields. Beyond Ramshorn Drive lies Allenwood and a welcoming general store with refreshments and trailside tables. Two consecutive pedestrian bridges leapfrog trail users over the roaring eight-lane Garden State Parkway. Then the trail transitions back into open farmland followed by a golf course and driving range.

The trail ends at Allaire State Park, where a world of diversions await: Tour historical Allaire Village for a look at a 19th-century iron-making community, or hop a ride on the antique cars of the steam-powered Pine Creek Railroad. The park provides additional hiking and biking trails, plus campsites if you need a little more time before rolling back to modern times on the Edgar Felix Memorial Bikeway.

DIRECTIONS

To reach the trail in Manasquan, take the Garden State Parkway to State Route 34 South. When you reach the traffic circle, take the third exit for State Route 524 East. Turn right on North Main Street in Manasquan; a municipal parking lot is on the left. The trail begins across the street from the parking lot.

From the Garden State Parkway, take the exit for New Jersey Route 138 East. Turn right onto Allenwood Road. Turn left onto 18th Avenue. Turn right onto Balleys Corner Road. Turn left onto Allaire Road (County Road 524). The entrance to the municipal complex is the first left.

To access the trail from Allaire State Park, from Interstate 195, take the exit for State Route 547 and Allaire State Park. Proceed north and turn right on State Route 524 toward Allaire State Park. Turn right on the park entrance road for the park office. The trail begins in the northeast corner of the large parking lot on the left.

Contact: Town of Manasquan
201 East Main Street
Manasquan, NJ 08736
(732) 223-0544
www.manasquan-nj.com

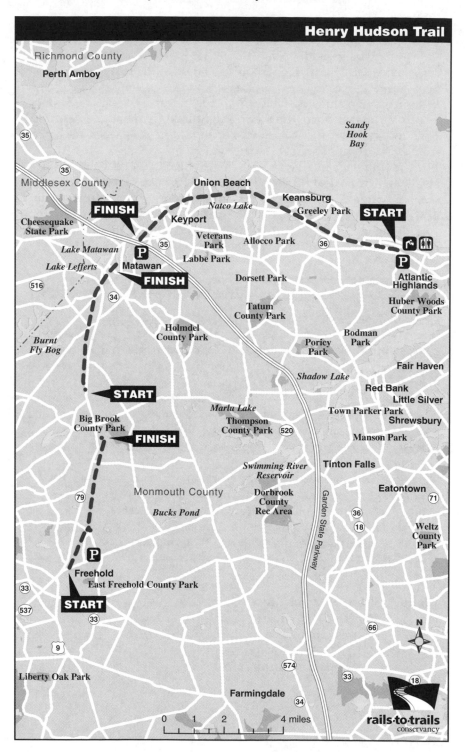

Henry Hudson Trail

Henry Hudson Trail

The Henry Hudson Trail is three trail segments along the same former railroad corridor. The gaps between the sections require significant on-road travel; it is best to consider them separate trails. You can choose from the 9.8-mile northern segment, 5-mile central segment, and 5-mile southern segment.

The longest and most scenic segment is the northern section. Arcing 9.8 miles from the Trail Activity Center Trailhead in Atlantic Highlands to Aberdeen, the Henry Hudson Trail traverses a trail-lined corridor and open saltwater marshes. The trail runs east and west on the north side of NJ Route 36 as it passes through residential neighborhoods. Wooden bridges cross marshlands and streams, and numerous residential street crossings require caution. Rabbits and chipmunks speed across the path, and the sky is filled with seagulls and a variety of songbirds. In approximately the middle of this northern segment an expansive marsh provides a view of the Manhattan skyline across Lower New York Bay.

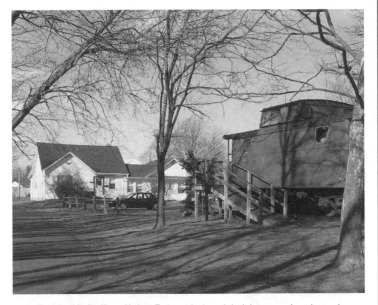

The relatively flat Henry Hudson Trail travels through both human-made and natural environments.

Location
Monmouth County

Endpoints
Avenue D and Highway 36 in Atlantic Highlands and Main Street/ NJ Route 537 in Freehold

Mileage
19.8

Roughness Index
1

Surface
Asphalt and dirt

Two 5-mile segments make up the southern reaches of the trail. A 2-mile separation between the two sections is designated for future trail construction. Starting at the Monmouth County Care Center in Freehold Township, the trail heads north through a wooded corridor in primarily residential suburban communities. Allen Avenue signals the end of this section in a residential neighborhood.

To reach the next trail section in Marlboro follow State Route 79 north. To reach Route 79 from Allen Avenue, follow Allen Avenue west to Maywood Drive. Turn right (north) on Maywood to Quincy Street and turn left (west). Follow Route 79 along the shoulder to Station Road on the left. Most of this segment is also wooded and passes through residential areas; it ends at Church Street in Matawan.

DIRECTIONS

To reach the Henry Hudson Trail Activity Center in Leonardo for the northern segment, take the Garden State Parkway to Exit 117. Follow Route 36 South toward Keyport for 9 miles. Use the Avenue D jughandle (all turns are from the right lane) for Route 36 North. Parking is marked at the Henry Hudson Activity Center.

To reach the intersection of Gerard Avenue and Clark Street in Keyport for the central section, head south on the Garden State Parkway and take Exit 117A. After the toll and at the first stop sign, turn left onto Lloyd Road. Cross over the parkway to the traffic light and turn left onto Gerard Avenue. The parking lot is on the right.

From the Garden State Parkway North take Exit 117. Bear right onto State Route 35 South to a U-turn on left. Travel back toward the Garden State Parkway entrance, and turn right before the toll plaza onto Clark Street. The parking lot is on the right after the traffic light.

To reach the Monmouth County Care Center for the southern segment, take the Garden State Parkway South to Exit 117A. After the toll, turn right at the stop sign onto Lloyd Road. Take Lloyd Road approximately 3 miles to Route 79 South. Continue on Route 79 South and turn left onto Kozloski Road, and continue approximately 7 miles. Turn right onto Dutch Lane Road. Monmouth County Care Center is on the right.

Contact: Monmouth County Park System
805 Newman Springs Road
Lincroft, NJ 07738
(732) 842-4000: Park System Headquarters
www.monmouthcountyparks.com

Kingston Branch Loop Trail

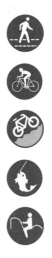

The Kingston Branch Loop Trail is a trip up one side and down the other of the scenic tree-lined Delaware and Raritan Canal. The eastern half of the loop follows the bed of the Rocky Hill Railroad and Transportation Company, which began operation between Kingston and Rocky Hill in 1870. The remainder of the loop travels the dirt and gravel canal towpath.

From the parking lot on the north side of State Route 27/Lincoln Highway, the crushed stone rail-trail travels 1.75 miles to State Route 518/Georgetown-Franklin Turnpike. Walk across the bridge over the canal on the narrow sidewalk, and turn left for the return trip south on the canal towpath.

The entire route is tree-lined and remains fairly cool on even the hottest summer days. With the peaceful Delaware and Raritan Canal in view at all times, you will bear witness to its popularity with boaters, birders and anglers. Canoes, kayaks and small craft with electric motors are permitted along this section of the

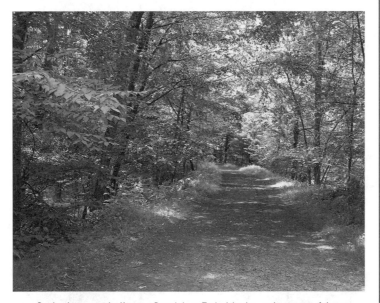

Catch a breeze on the Kingston Branch Loop Trail while also catching views of the Delaware and Raritan Canal as you cycle along.

Location
Somerset County

Endpoints
Route 27/Lincoln Highway in Kingston

Mileage
3.7

Roughness Index
2

Surface
Dirt, crushed stone and gravel

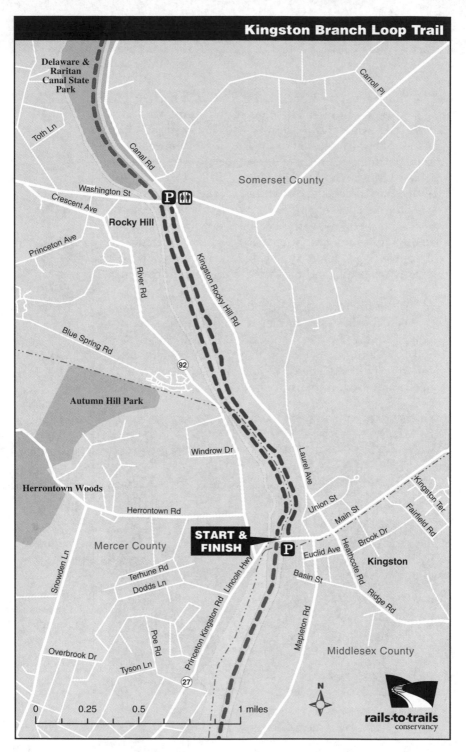

Kingston Branch Loop Trail

Delaware & Raritan Canal State Park

Carroll Pl

Toth Ln

Canal Rd

Somerset County

Washington St

Crescent Ave

Rocky Hill

Princeton Ave

River Rd

Kingston Rocky Hill Rd

Blue Spring Rd

92

Autumn Hill Park

Windrow Dr

Herrontown Woods

Laurel Ave

Herrontown Rd

Union St

Main St

Kingston Ter

Fairfield Rd

Mercer County

START & FINISH

Euclid Ave

Heathcote Rd

Brook Dr

Kingston

Snowden Ln

Terhune Rd

Dodds Ln

Princeton Kingston Rd

Lincoln Hwy

Basin St

Mapleton Rd

Ridge Rd

Middlesex County

Overbrook Dr

Poe Rd

Tyson Ln

27

0   0.25   0.5   1 miles

N

rails·to·trails
conservancy

watered canal. Bass, sunfish, perch and annually stocked trout are just some of the fish in the canal.

On your way back to the trailhead on Route 27, take time to explore the restored Lock #8, the locktender's house and the site of an old mill. The charming village of Kingston contains five historic districts worth exploring for an afternoon.

DIRECTIONS

From US Route 1 take Ridge Road west to Kingston. At the State Route 27 traffic light turn left. Proceed approximately a quarter mile, and turn right into the parking lot.

Contact: D&R Canal State Park
145 Mapleton Road
Princeton, NJ 08540
(609) 924-5705
www.dandrcanal.com/gen_info.html#trails

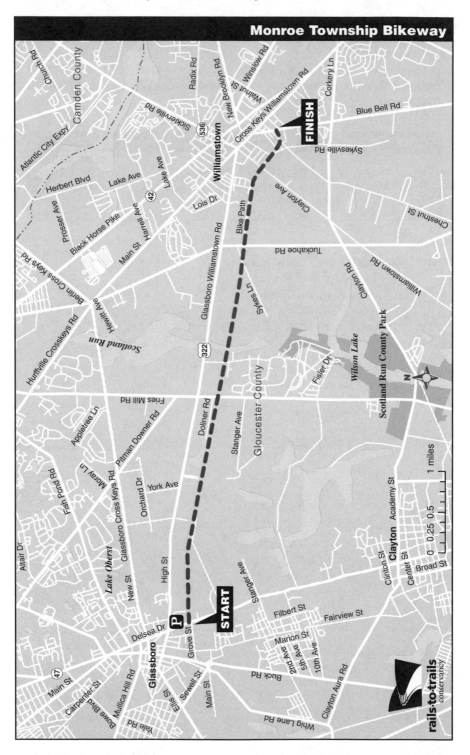

Monroe Township Bikeway

Monroe Township Bikeway

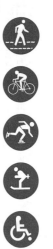

The Monroe Township Bikeway is a 6.25-mile connection between the suburban communities of Glassboro and Williamstown. The trail through Glassboro passes through the dense forest of the Glassboro Fish and Wildlife Management Area, and then transitions through quiet residential neighborhoods and community open spaces. The trail follows the former right-of-way of the Pennsylvania-Reading Seashore Line that served the New Jersey shore points of Atlantic City, Ocean City, Wildwood and Cape May. The Seashore Line did not follow a stream valley like so many eastern rail corridors; the result is a trail that is arrow straight for long distances.

Beginning in Glassboro the trail cuts east and passes a few commercial and industrial properties before it enters a hardwood forest within the Glassboro Fish and Wildlife Management Area. The heavy tree canopy helps keep this section of the trail cooler during summer.

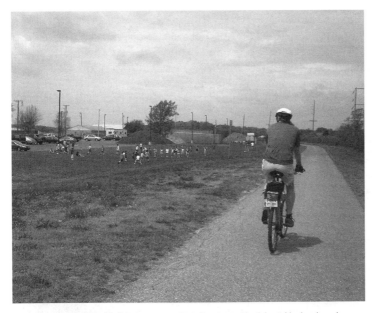

The Monroe Township Bikeway passes through quiet residential neighborhoods and community open spaces.

Location
Gloucester County

Endpoints
Delsea Drive (Route 47) in Glassboro to Blue Bell Road in Williamstown

Mileage
6.25

Roughness Index
1

Surface
Asphalt

25

The forest thins out to a single-file line of trees on both sides before crossing Monroe Avenue. After the street crossing, the trail returns to a heavily wooded forest for the next mile and a half.

The bikeway emerges from the forest at the edge of a residential neighborhood. The route becomes more open as it passes residential neighborhoods for about a half mile before returning to forested shade. After crossing North Tuckahoe Road, you pass the Williamstown Middle School complex with ball fields and a football stadium. The trail crosses Clayton Road and runs parallel to Railroad Avenue for a short distance, and you pass community ball fields.

The trail reaches an unassuming end at Blue Bell Road across the street from the Williamstown Police Station. A plaque at the Williamstown end of the bikeway designates it as the George F. McDonald Sr. Memorial Bike Path. McDonald served as mayor of Williamstown from 1975 to 1978. A convenience store at the end of the trail is perfect for stocking up on refreshments before returning to Glassboro.

DIRECTIONS

To reach the western end, from US Route 322 in Glassboro, turn south onto State Route 47/Delsea Drive. Bike route signs along Route 47 point to the start of the trail. There is very limited public parking at this location along the entrance road to a housing development.

To reach the eastern end, from US Route 322 in Williamstown, take Clayton Road south. Turn left on Railroad Avenue, which becomes Ames Road. The start of the trail is near the intersection of Ames Road and Chestnut Street. The Williamstown end of the trail has even less public parking than Glassboro.

Contact: Township of Monroe, Gloucester County
125 Virginia Avenue
Williamstown, NJ 08094
(856) 728-9800
www.monroetownshipnj.org

Paulinskill Valley Trail

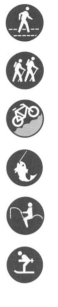

For a dose of rural scenery head to the northwest corner of New Jersey where this 27-mile rail-trail cuts a nearly uninterrupted path along the banks of the Paulins Kill, a Delaware River tributary that gives the trail its name. (*Kill* is from the Dutch and refers to a creek; it is used in areas of New Jersey, New York, Pennsylvania and Delaware). Farms line the corridor; you are likely to be in the company of equestrians, bicyclists and hikers. When the snow flies, skiers, snowshoers and even dog sled teams hit the route. There are occasional hints of the railroad that carried coal, produce and dairy products to points east on the corridor. Look for the original railroad mileage posts.

From the trailhead in Knowlton Township, several miles east of the Delaware River, the trail travels east along the north side of the Paulins Kill. In about a mile you pass under the massive Paulinskill Viaduct, also know as the Hainsburg Viaduct, an impressive

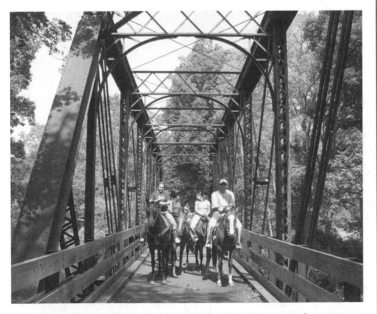

While on the Paulinskill Valley Trail, you are likely to be in the company of equestrians, bicyclists and hikers.

Location
Sussex and Warren counties

Endpoints
Brugler Road in Knowlton Township to Sparta Junction in Sussex County

Mileage
27

Roughness Index
3

Surface
Cinder, dirt and grass

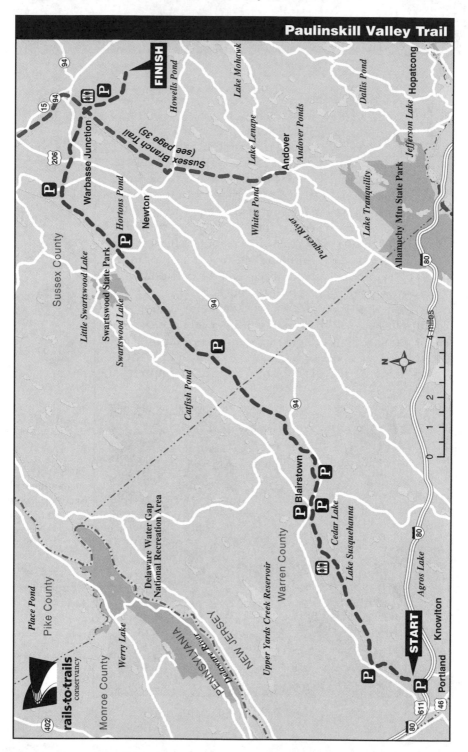

Paulinskill Valley Trail

structure built by the Delaware, Lackawanna and Western Railroad in 1910. With seven arches reaching 115 feet up and stretching 1,100 feet from end to end, the viaduct was the world's largest reinforced concrete structure in its time.

At about mile 5, the trail passes through the Blairstown Airport, known for its glider rides over the Kittatinny Mountain Ridge. A runway restaurant with picnic tables provides front-row viewing of the planes and gliders. Lake Susquehanna is just to the south of the trail.

In Blairstown Township, Footbridge Park is a good spot for taking a break or exploring the town. A large parking area makes this an informal trailhead for the rail-trail.

The trail crosses the Paulinskill several times over the next 4.5 miles. Upon reaching Stillwater Road, the stream and the trail diverge and the trail enters a wooded wetland.

Just before Paulinskill Lake the route is interrupted by a missing bridge. A side path descends from the corridor to the road below. After crossing Sussex County Route 614, the path ascends back up to the railroad grade. Back on the trail you get an elevated view of the long skinny lake and the cottages that line its shores. Another bridge has been removed 2.25 miles farther at NJ Route 622. As before you must descend from the trail to the road and then climb back up to the elevated rail corridor. Exercise caution using these unmaintained side paths.

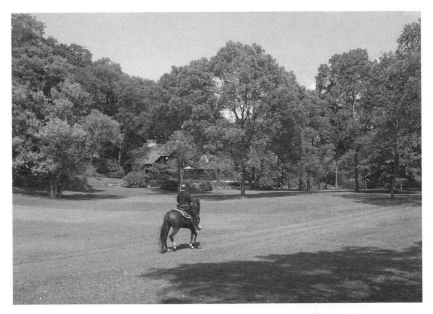

Upon reaching Stillwater Road, the trail diverges from the stream and enters a wooded wetland.

When the trail enters the Paulinskill Wildlife Management Area, near Paulins Kill Lake wildlife abounds. You may encounter wild turkey, white-tailed deer, and numerous species of birds and ducks as you make your way through the hardwood forests and wetlands.

Don't miss this connection: The Sussex Branch Trail (see page 35) intersects the Paulinskill Valley Trail in Warbasse Junction. A trailhead near this junction provides parking and a restroom on NJ Route 663.

Beyond this point the trail is not well maintained, so be prepared for what could be an adventure. The remaining 0.6 mile includes several stream crossings with narrow footbridges. This part of the trail is little used and not maintained so it may be overgrown and blocked by fallen trees or vegetation. The right-of-way ends abruptly at an active rail corridor. There is no public road access here.

DIRECTIONS

To reach the Station Road Trailhead in Knowltown Township, from Interstate 80 take the Columbia exit and follow State Route 94 east. Turn right on Station Road. The trailhead is on the right side of the road just past the stone arch bridge.

To reach the northeastern endpoint north of Newton, from Newton take US Route 206/State Route 94 north. Bear right and continue on Route 94. Turn right onto Warbasse Junction Road. The trailhead will be on your left.

Contact: Kittatinny Valley State Park
P.O. Box 621
Andover, NJ 07821
(973) 786-6445
www.nj.gov/dep/parksandforests/parks/kittval.html

Paulinskill Valley Trail Committee
P.O. Box 175
Andover, NJ 07821
(908) 684-4820
www.pvtc-kvsp.org/

Pleasantville to Somers Point Bike Path

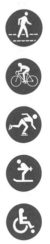

This is a true community trail: Four small cities are tied together by this 6.5-mile corridor, each maintaining their short section and calling it a different name. Starting in Somers Point, a few blocks from the Atlantic Ocean, a large bright sign welcomes you to the SOMERS POINT BICYCLE PATH. The trail then heads north through Linwood, Northfield and Pleasantville. Atlantic City is about a dozen miles northeast, and the area leans toward an urban setting. Frequent street crossings require caution.

Most of the trail travels through residential neighborhoods and the schools, parks and playing fields in between. Students use the path as a safe walking route from home to school. Residents of the trail's neighborhoods frequently walk it for exercise or take their babies for a ride along it in a stroller. Lightly traveled neighborhood roads—and busier Shore Road to the east—parallel much of the bike path, so a meal is never far away. A

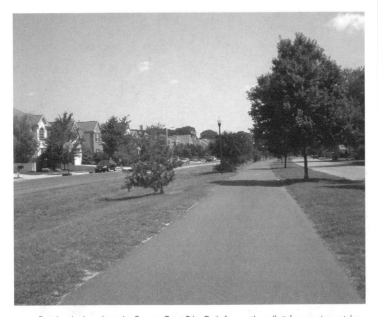

People who live along the Somers Point Bike Path frequently walk it for exercise or take their babies along for a ride.

Location
Atlantic County

Endpoints
West New Jersey Avenue and 1st Avenue in Somers Point to West Decatur Avenue in Pleasantville

Mileage
6.5

Roughness Index
1

Surface
Asphalt

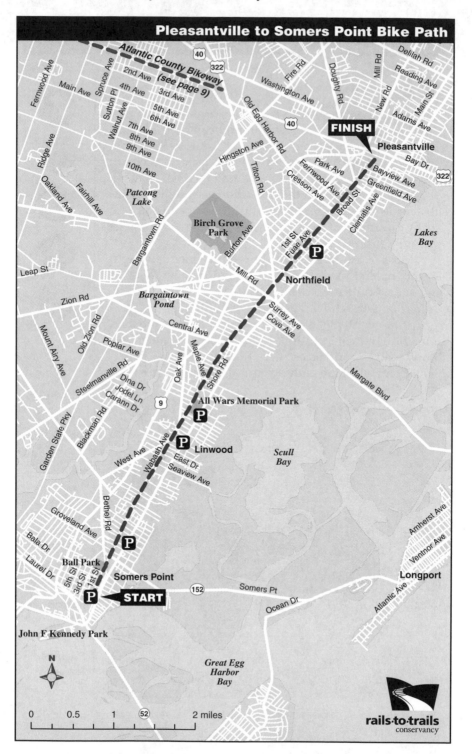

few short wooded sections provide a change of pace from the residential neighborhoods that make up most of the path's viewscape.

From the municipal building in Somers Point at the intersection of West New Jersey Avenue and 1st Street, the bike path heads north parallel to 1st Street, passing areas of primarily commercial properties. Beyond Maryland Avenue the area on either side of the bike path is primarily residential.

Just after passing over Ocean Avenue, the bike path enters Linwood (and is occasionally the Linwood Bike Path), which consists primarily of residential neighborhoods. The bike path takes the center of a wide median that divides Wabash Avenue, the eastern side is one way north and the western side is one way south.

The bikeway enters Northfield just prior to crossing Oakhurst Avenue. More residential neighborhoods flank the bikeway. A large recreational complex provides ample parking trailside between West Devonshire and Edgewood Avenues.

Enter Pleasantville, the most urban of the communities, after passing over West Ridgewood Avenue. The trail continues to West Decatur Avenue and extends across the inactive railroad bridge that crosses the Black Horse Pike.

DIRECTIONS

To reach Somers Point, from US Routes 322/40 (Black Horse Pike) take US Route 9/New Road South 2.2 miles. Turn left on West Mill Road. Turn right on Shore Road and go 4.3 miles. Turn right onto West New Jersey Avenue. Turn right onto 1st Avenue. Parking is on the right.

To reach Pleasantville, US Routes 322/40 (Black Horse Pike) in the town becomes West Verona Avenue. Turn right onto South Main Street. Proceed one block and turn right onto Decatur Avenue. There is limited curbside parking.

Contact: Somers Point
Community, Education and Recreation Office
1 West New Jersey Avenue
Somers Point, NJ 08244
(609) 927-5253
www.somerspointgov.org

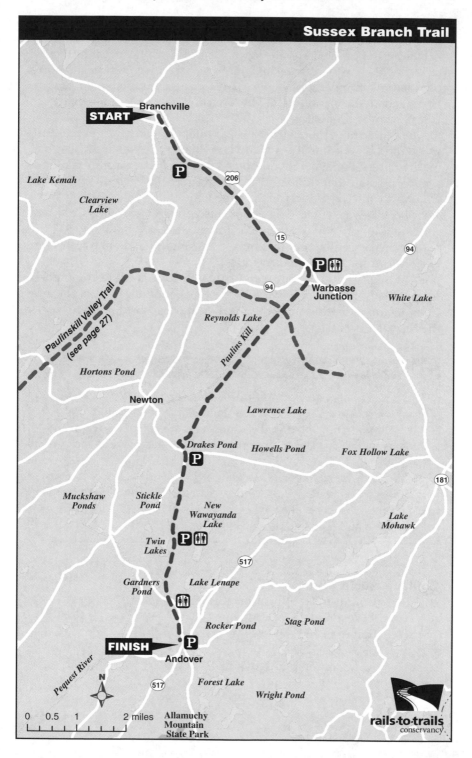

Sussex Branch Trail

START — Branchville

P

206

15

94

94

P 🛉🛉 Warbasse Junction

White Lake

Lake Kemah

Clearview Lake

Paulinskill Valley Trail (see page 27)

Reynolds Lake

Paulins Kill

Hortons Pond

Newton

Lawrence Lake

Drakes Pond

P

Howells Pond

Fox Hollow Lake

181

Muckshaw Ponds

Stickle Pond

New Wawayanda Lake

Lake Mohawk

Twin Lakes

P 🛉🛉

517

Gardners Pond

Lake Lenape

🛉🛉

Rocker Pond

Stag Pond

FINISH —

P

Andover

Pequest River

N

517

Forest Lake

Wright Pond

0   0.5   1   2 miles

Allamuchy Mountain State Park

rails·to·trails
conservancy

Sussex Branch Trail

The Sussex Branch Trail got its start in the late 1840s as the narrow-gauge, mule-drawn Sussex Mine Railroad, whose primary purpose was hauling iron ore from the mines in Andover to Waterloo Village on the Morris Canal. The railroad was eventually upgraded and expanded before being merged into the Delaware, Lackawanna and Western Railroad in the mid-1940s. Though the railroad was out of service several decades later, the state of New Jersey—which owns much of the area parkland—preserved the right-of-way for trail use.

The trail begins on the outskirts of Branchville at a parking area along Augusta Hill Road. (The trail extends about a mile north from this location, but limited access and parking make this the best jumping-off point.) The Sussex Branch Trail is generally oriented north and south while the Paulinskill Valley Trail (see

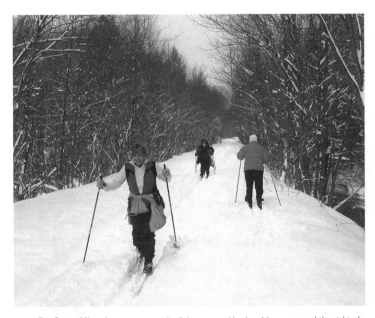

The State of New Jersey owns much of the area parkland and has preserved the right-of-way for trail use.

Location
Sussex County

Endpoints
Mill Street in Branchville to Smith Street in Byram Township

Mileage
13.4

Roughness Index
3

Surface
Cinder, dirt and grass

page 27), which it intersects at Warbasse Junction, is generally oriented east and west.

The trail hugs the banks of the Paulinskill River, and a series of bridges cross the stream. After crossing County Route 565 the trail runs parallel with NJ Route 15 into the historic village of Lafayette. Antique shops and the Olde Lafayette Village outlet shops line Route 15.

From here the Sussex Branch Trail travels through fairly dense forest until Warbasse Junction where it meets the Paulinskill Valley Trail. Only 300 feet west along the Paulinskill Valley Trail from the intersection is a trailhead with parking and restroom facilities.

A break in the trail corridor requires on-road travel for 1.1 miles. A large sign just north of Newton directs trail users to Route 663/ Hicks Avenue. This tree-lined, two-lane road has limited narrow shoulders that require extra caution. The trail resumes on the south side of Hicks Avenue near the intersection with Sparta Avenue.

Kittatinny Valley State Park is a highlight of this trail. The park's maples, hickories and tulip poplars contribute to a riot of fall color. In spring, wildflowers flourish and flowering trees and shrubs brighten the park's glacially formed valleys and limestone ridges. Birders flock to the park to view some of the 200 bird species spotted in the area, and hikers and mountain bikers seek their thrill on a network of trails throughout the park.

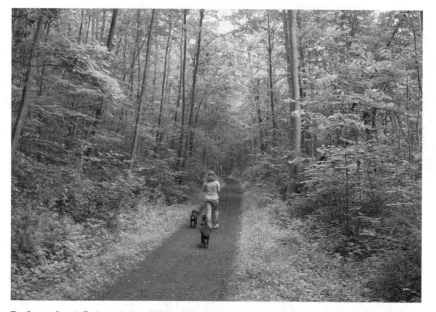

The Sussex Branch Trail travels through fairly dense forest until it meets Warbasse Junction at the Paulinskill Valley Trail.

The town of Andover with eateries and shops lies on the south side of the state park, after crossing US Route 206. The parking area at the intersection of Smith Street and Railroad Avenue is a good point to end your trip. The trail is 13.3 miles long to this point. The remaining 5 miles of corridor to Waterloo Road becomes difficult to follow as it passes through residential areas, along the side of US Route 206 and around Cranberry Lake before entering Allamuchy Mountain State Park.

DIRECTIONS

From Branchville, proceed south on US Route 206. Turn right onto Augusta Hill Road. The trailhead will be on your right.

To reach Andover, from Interstate 80, take US Route 206 north. In Andover, turn left onto Brighton Avenue. Turn right onto Railroad Avenue. Parking is at the intersection of Smith Street and Railroad Avenue.

To reach Kittatinny Valley State Park in Andover, from Route 80, take Route 206 north approximately 8 miles through Andover Borough. Turn right onto Goodale Road and follow it approximately 1 mile to the park entrance on the right.

Contact: Kittatinny Valley State Park
P. O. Box 621
Andover, NJ 07821
(973) 786-6445
www.nj.gov/dep/parksandforests/parks/kittval.html

Paulinskill Valley Trail Committee
P.O. Box 175
Andover, NJ 07821
(908) 684-4820
www.pvtc-kvsp.org/

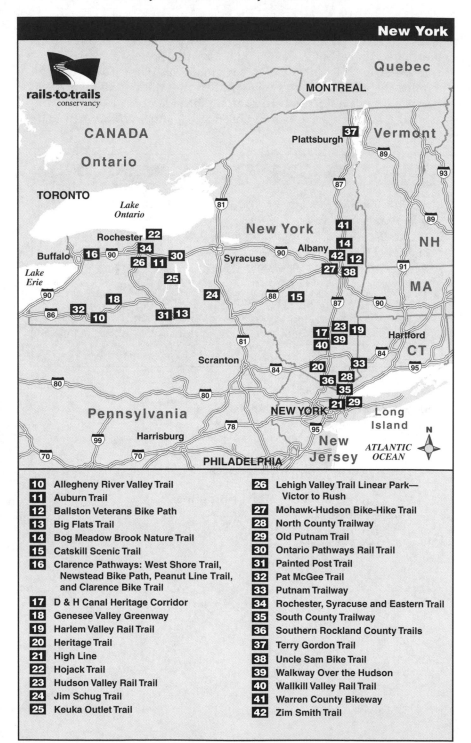

New York

rails·to·trails
conservancy

Quebec

MONTREAL

CANADA

Plattsburgh **37** Vermont

Ontario

89

93

TORONTO

87

Lake
Ontario

81

89

New York **41**

Rochester **22**

Albany **14**

NH

Buffalo **16** **90** **34**

30

Syracuse **90**

42 **12**

26 **11**

27 **38**

91

Lake
Erie

25

MA

90

18

24

88 **15**

87

90

32

86

10

31 **13**

17 **23** **19**

Hartford

40 **39**

81

CT

Scranton

20 **33**

84

84

95

80

36 **28**

80

35

Pennsylvania

NEW YORK

21 **29**

Long
Island

78

N

99

Harrisburg

95

New

ATLANTIC

70

70

PHILADELPHIA

Jersey

OCEAN

10 Allegheny River Valley Trail		**26** Lehigh Valley Trail Linear Park—	
11 Auburn Trail		Victor to Rush	
12 Ballston Veterans Bike Path		**27** Mohawk-Hudson Bike-Hike Trail	
13 Big Flats Trail		**28** North County Trailway	
14 Bog Meadow Brook Nature Trail		**29** Old Putnam Trail	
15 Catskill Scenic Trail		**30** Ontario Pathways Rail Trail	
16 Clarence Pathways: West Shore Trail,		**31** Painted Post Trail	
Newstead Bike Path, Peanut Line Trail,		**32** Pat McGee Trail	
and Clarence Bike Trail		**33** Putnam Trailway	
17 D & H Canal Heritage Corridor		**34** Rochester, Syracuse and Eastern Trail	
18 Genesee Valley Greenway		**35** South County Trailway	
19 Harlem Valley Rail Trail		**36** Southern Rockland County Trails	
20 Heritage Trail		**37** Terry Gordon Trail	
21 High Line		**38** Uncle Sam Bike Trail	
22 Hojack Trail		**39** Walkway Over the Hudson	
23 Hudson Valley Rail Trail		**40** Wallkill Valley Rail Trail	
24 Jim Schug Trail		**41** Warren County Bikeway	
25 Keuka Outlet Trail		**42** Zim Smith Trail	

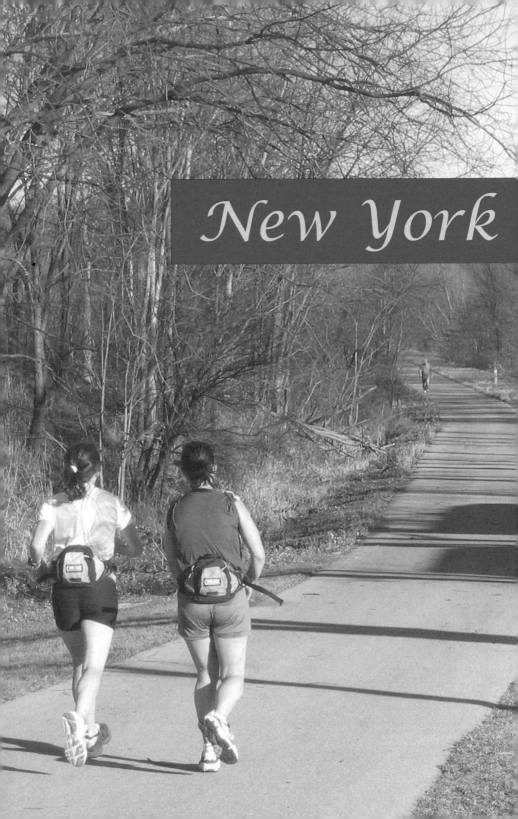

New York

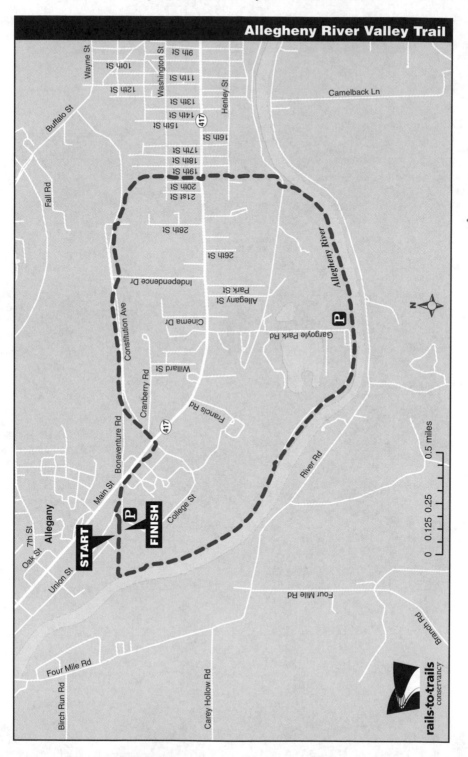

Allegheny River Valley Trail

Allegheny River Valley Trail

If you find yourself in Allegany or Olean, New York, with a half hour to spare, this loop trail makes for a very enjoyable bike ride. Better yet, strap on your inline skates and do a lap or two with the other skaters, bicyclists, walkers, baby-jogger parents and training-wheel children who flock to this pleasant trail.

Where a typical rail bed is stick straight, this 5.6-mile circular route winds and dips along a river valley. Its rail-trail designation comes from the active railroad that runs adjacent to the corridor for a short distance on the north side. There are 115 such rail-with-trail facilities in the nation.

The southern half of the trail is on the Allegheny River, and the rest of the loop has many access points in the small communities of Allegany and Olean. Starting near the tennis courts of St. Bonaventure University and heading west brings you to the river quickly. The trail encircles the school, making it popular with students

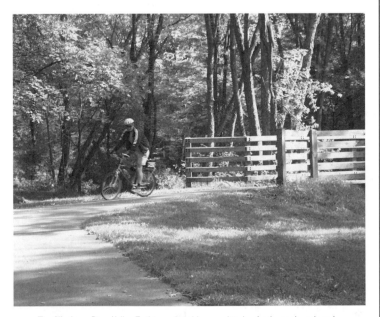

The Allegheny River Valley Trail is enclosed by a multitude of oak, maple, ash and cherry trees.

Location
Cattaraugus County

Endpoint
St. Bonaventure University

Mileage
5.6

Roughness Index
1

Surface
Asphalt

who use it for recreation. A leafy tree canopy cools off summer days and, in winter, lets in warming sunshine. At the first bend, the trail descends a little and the river comes into view. Oaks, maples, ash, and cherry trees enclose the trail. In first 2 miles a few well-designed small bridges carry you over small tributaries to the river and the trail becomes slightly wider. Another slight descent followed by a curve at mile 1.5 warrants the trail's 15 miles per hour speed limit. Be watchful for oncoming traffic.

At mile 2 the river widens and you reach Gargoyle Park, with parking, swings, and plenty of room for children who have been in a buggy or bike seat to run around. Large shagbark hickory trees—with distinctive gray shaggy bark—dominate the park grounds. Soon after the park, the trail crosses a small stream on another bridge.

When you reach the levee restraining the Allegheny River, you have gone 3 miles. Although it's unpaved, the levee is used as a bike and running path, adding more miles to the local trail system. Soon after the levee you enter a residential area and cross a few streets, including West State Street (Route 417). Use caution on this long, busy road crossing. The corridor soon widens and is shared with telephone lines and underground gas lines. After crossing Constitution Avenue, the trail passes several shops, including an ice cream stand popular with students.

The Olean rail yard, at mile 4, marks where the trail parallels freight train tracks for a quarter mile. The rail yard inspired Joe Higgins, a local resident credited with dreaming up the trail. As Higgins visited rail-trails in Rhode Island, Vermont and California, his idea for the circular rail-with-trail took shape. He helped negotiate a lease agreement among the communities, landowners and state Department of Transportation, which provided funding for the trail.

In front of the university the trail crosses back over Route 417, turns right, continues for another half mile along the road or sidewalk, and reaches the tennis court parking lot where you can wind down your adventure. If you still have energy, take another lap on this excellent trail.

DIRECTIONS

To reach St. Bonaventure University from Allegheny, from Interstate 86 take Exit 24. Turn south on Five Mile Road and then immediately left onto Route 417. Proceed a little more than 1 mile until you cross a railroad overpass and see St. Bonaventure University on your right. Make the first right into the campus and another immediate right. Before you cross the railroad tracks again, turn left on an unmarked uphill street. After 50 yards you will see the trailhead and parking lot on your right before the tennis courts.

Gargoyle Park is another entrance off Route 417 and usually less congested. Go a quarter mile past the entrance to the university and turn right on Gargoyle Park Road.

Contact: Greater Olean Area Chamber of Commerce
120 North Union Street
Olean, NY 14760
(716) 372-4433
www.allegany.org/index.php?alleganytowntrail

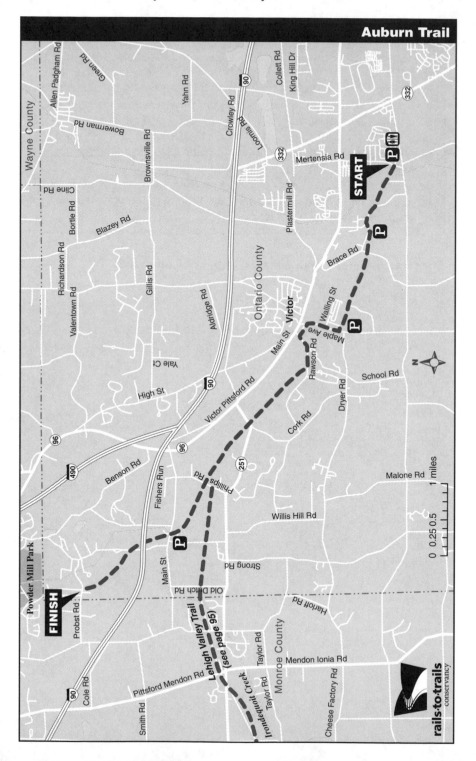

Auburn Trail

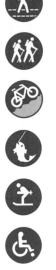

The Auburn Trail is a major cross-town multi-use pathway. Work to improve the trail and extend it to Powder Mill Park is underway, but for now there are several short detours on area roads. The trail makes up for the inconvenience by providing connections with other trails and an up-close view of one of the oldest railroad buildings in the country.

Start the ride in Farmington at Mertensia Park. Shortly after leaving the park, the trail passes through a residential development. At Victor Road (approximately 0.75 mile) you encounter your first detour. Follow Victor Road to Break of Day Road to a left turn onto Brace Road and back to the rail corridor. The detour is about 0.9 mile long on lightly trafficked residential streets.

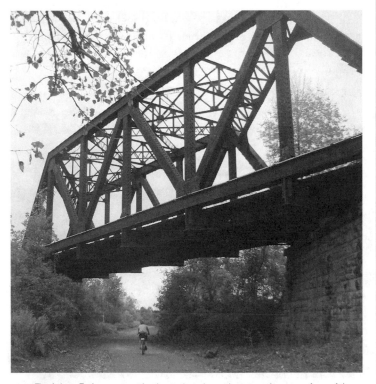

The Auburn Trail connects with other trails and provides an up-close view of one of the oldest railroad buildings in the country.

Location
Ontario County

Endpoints
Mertensia Park in Farmington to Railroad Mills Road in Victor

Mileage
9.1

Roughness Index
2

Surface
Cinder, dirt and grass

Back on the trail, Victor Hills Golf Club is on the left. A little farther along, a restored train station and boxcars have been repurposed for business use. Just past these landmarks is the second and last on-road detour. Turn right on Maple Street, cross the railroad tracks and turn left onto Railroad Avenue. After one block, turn left onto School Street to return to the trail. To explore the shops and restaurants in the village of Victor, stay straight on Maple Street one block beyond Railroad Avenue until you reach Main Street.

The trail is much more rural beyond Victor. Seneca Trail, a 7.5-mile hiking trail, branches off right. In another 1.8 miles the trail passes under the Lehigh Valley Trail (see page 95). To significantly boost your mileage follow the Lehigh Valley Trail 15 miles west to the Genesee Valley Greenway (see page 67).

Next up on the Auburn Trail is Fishers, where the trail cuts through the parking lot of the Fishers Fire Company and passes the second oldest railroad feature in the U.S.—a cobblestone pumping station. The station supplied water to the steam engines that traveled this line from 1841, when the Auburn and Rochester Railroad began operation, through the 1853 consolidation into the New York Central Railroad.

The trail corridor continues more than 2 miles from Fishers to Powder Mill Park. This section is not yet formally developed, but hikers and sturdy cyclists will find it passable. A large railroad tunnel whisks you under the New York State Thruway before you arrive at the trail's end at Probst Road.

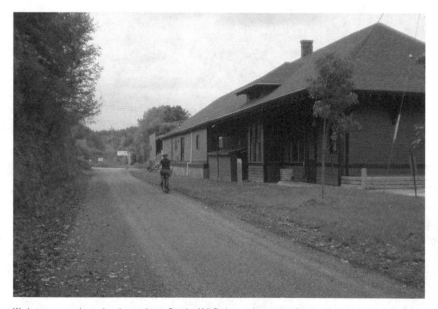

Work to improve the trail and extend it to Powder Mill Park is underway, but for now there are several short detours on area roads.

DIRECTIONS

To reach Mertensia Park in Farmington, from Interstate 90 (New York State Thruway) exit onto State Route 332 South. Go approximately 1.5 miles to State Route 96 (Victor-Manchester Road) turn right. After about a half mile turn left on Mertensia Road. Trail parking, at Mertensia Park, is on the right.

To reach Maple Avenue in Victor, from Interstate 90 (New York State Thruway) exit onto State Route 332 South. Go approximately 1.5 miles to State Route 96 (Victor-Manchester Road), and turn right. After 1.9 miles turn left onto Main Street in Victor. Turn left onto Maple Avenue in about 0.7 mile. Parking is on the right at the former railroad station.

To reach Main Street in Fishers, from Interstate 90 (New York State Thruway) exit onto State Route 332 South. Go approximately 1.5 miles to State Route 96 (Victor-Manchester Road) turn right. After 1.9 miles turn left onto Main Street in Victor, which becomes Victor-Pittsford Road. In about 4 miles turn left onto Main Street in Fishers. Parking is on the left behind the fire station.

Contact: Victor Hiking Trails, Inc.
85 East Main Street
Victor, NY 14564
(585) 234-8226
www.victorhikingtrails.org

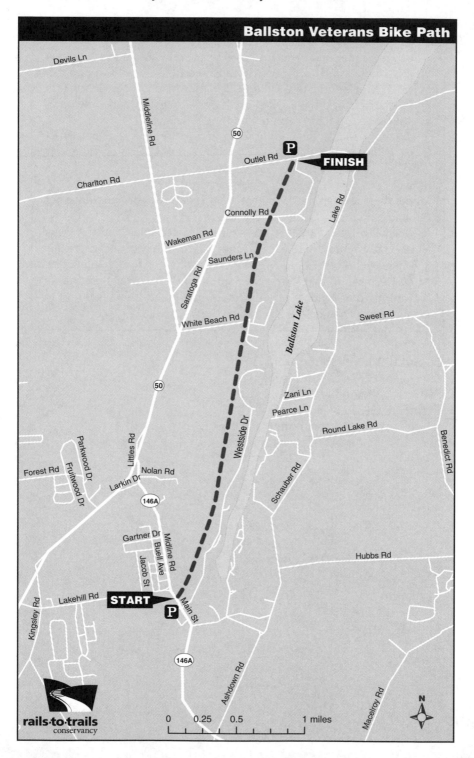

Ballston Veterans Bike Path

Ballston Veterans Bike Path

This asphalt trail is the legacy of an interurban trolley system operated by Schenectady Railway Company (SRC) in the early 1900s. To attract visitors on weekends, SRC built an amusement park at Ballston Lake with a beachfront, some baseball fields, and oval tracks for bike races and footraces. Passengers paid 25 cents to ride the wooden trolley car from Schenectady to Ballston Lake and beyond, even to Saratoga Springs. The trolley ceased operation in 1940, and the amusement park is just a memory now. There's good bass fishing, however, at the fishing pier on Ballston Lake, not far from the Outlet Road Trailhead.

The Ballston Veterans Bike Path has a lot to offer. Informative signs fill you in on the trail corridor's history. Every quarter mile, mileage markers help you track your progress. The trail is conveniently reached from New York 146A, a main route into town. The bike

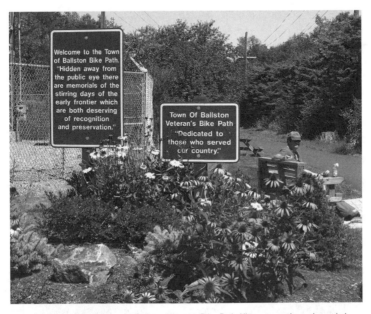

Informative signs along the Ballston Veterans Bike Path fill you in on the trail corridor's history, and mileage markers every quarter mile help you track your progress.

Location
Saratoga County

Endpoints
NY Route 146A to Outlet Road and Powers Lane in Ballston Lake

Length
3.5

Roughness Index
1

Surface
Asphalt

path will some day link up with an emerging network of multi-use trails in Saratoga County.

At the trailhead on Main Street watch for a monument dedicated to veterans from the town. Trees border much of the trail on your left, giving way for a time to scrub growth that allows a pleasing view of pastures and woods beyond. To the right, a berm with sumac, holly and other shrubs separates the path from an active rail line. The Canadian Pacific tracks parallel the trail for most of its length. The path is open overhead—don't forget sunscreen.

Parking at Outlet Road is limited. Across the road, the trolley corridor—overgrown—appears to continue. For now, however, you'll need to retrace your route back to the start. If you brought your fishing rod and license, however, go right on Outlet Road and look for the sign for the fishing pier.

DIRECTIONS

For the Route 146A Trailhead, take Exit 9 off Interstate 87 and head west on State Route 146. Take Route 146A north for about 6.5 miles to the Village of Ballston Lake. Shortly after crossing the railroad tracks, you'll spot the parking area for the bike path on your right.

Contact: Town of Ballston
323 Charlton Road
Ballston Spa, NY 12020
(518) 885-8502, extension 10
www.townofballstonny.org

Big Flats Trail

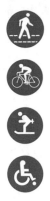

A pleasant walk between wetland habitat and farmland, this short community trail sits atop a sewer line that Corning Glassworks installed to serve its Big Flats plant. Corning provided the crushed stone surface for the trail.

The main trailhead is located near the center of the path off Kahler Road. A lovely new park with a pond, nature trail and a picnic pavilion is located here. It was developed by community volunteers in tribute to New York State Trooper Andrew J. Sperr who was killed in the line of duty by suspected bank robbers. The park was designed as a continuation of the Lowes Pond wetland area.

Heading west from the trailhead, the trail descends briefly and then flattens out for about a mile. Wetlands on both sides of the trail make this a great place to observe the variety of birdlife here. The trail ends at Winters

Location
Chemung County

Endpoints
Kahler Road to
Hibbard Road in
Elmira

Mileage
1.7

Roughness Index
2

Surface
Gravel

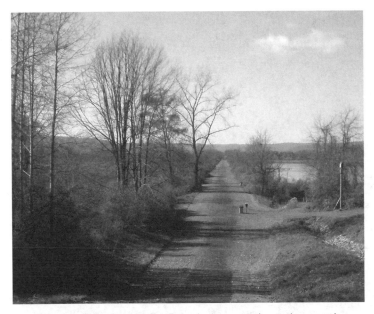

Wetlands on both sides of Big Flats Trail make this a great place to observe a wide variety of birdlife.

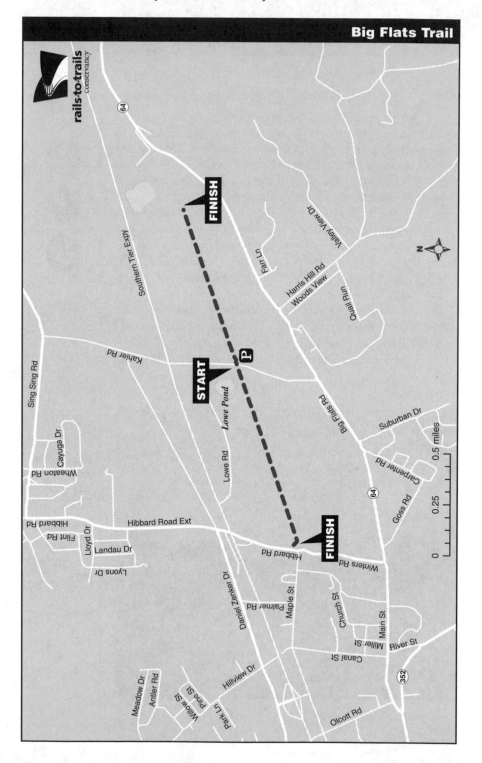

Big Flats Trail

Road in a residential neighborhood. This entire section of the trail is open wetlands and doesn't provide much shade.

East from the Kahler Road Trailhead is a more shaded experience. Woods on one side of the trail and a line of trees on the other keep you under leafy cover. The line of trees separates you from cultivated farmland until the trail dead-ends just before reaching Big Flats Road/County Route 64. There is no easy access to the road from this location.

A local transportation council has recommended that the Big Flats Rail Trail be better connected to Consumer Square Mall and Big Flats Town Center, and also extend to the Town of Horseheads, connecting it with the Catharine Valley Trail. If these extensions are made, this trail will become more than a pleasant place to walk or bike—it will be a useful transportation connection for the community.

DIRECTIONS

From Interstate 86 in Elmira, take Exit 50 onto Route 63 South, also Kahler Road. Follow approximately a quarter mile to park entrance. The trailhead is on the right.

Contact: Big Flats Department of Public Works
476 Maple Street
Big Flats, NY 14814
(607) 562-8443, extension 224
www.bigflatsny.gov

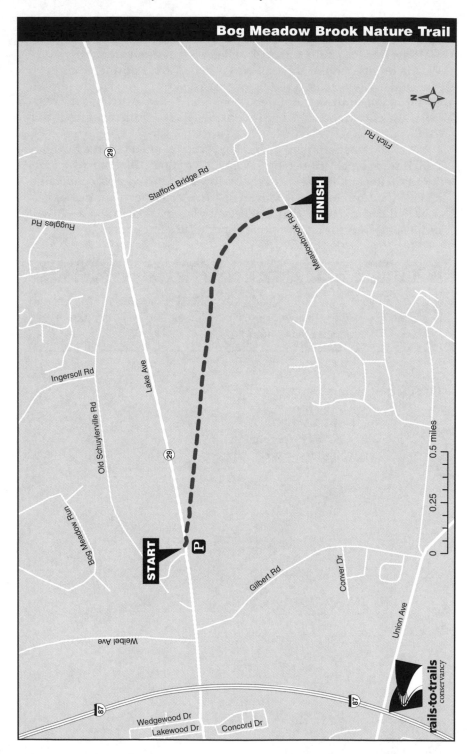

Bog Meadow Brook Nature Trail

T his out-and-back rail-trail's beautiful natural setting and informative signage invite visitors to
appreciate the importance of wetland habitats.
Located just east of downtown Saratoga Springs, the
trail allows you to observe and learn about three distinct types of wetland: open marsh, wet meadow (with
grasses, shrubs and small trees) and forested wetland
(lush with moss and ferns among the trees). Kids may
want to bring a fishing pole and drop a line from the
bridge.

Enjoying all this wetland comes at a cost. Portions
of the trail may be damp even in dry weather, and after
a heavy rain the trail can be downright messy. Think of
it this way: The soft surface makes it easier to spot tracks
of deer and other animals that have crossed the trail.

The initial half mile, from the start at Route 29, is
smooth sailing. The trail is level and suitable for wheelchair use. For much of the rest of the trail, however,

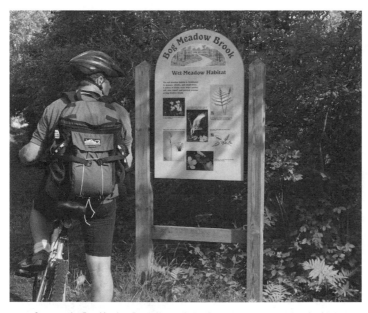

Signs on the Bog Meadow Brook Nature Trail explain the importance of wetland habitats.

Location
Saratoga County

Endpoints
Route 29 to
Meadowbrook Road
in Saratoga Springs

Mileage
2

**Roughness
Index**
3

Surface
Ballast and dirt

55

railroad ties remain visibly in place, making an uneven trail surface that is challenging even with a mountain bike. Pay attention to the posted warning that yellow jackets nest in the rotting railroad ties underfoot. If you have a bee-sting allergy, come prepared with emergency supplies.

At about mile 1.5 a handsome wooden boardwalk spans open marsh. The boardwalk and its benches provide a rare opportunity to be surrounded by wetlands while keeping your feet dry.

The trail is maintained by volunteers of Saratoga P.L.A.N. (Preserving Land and Nature). The organization provides a trail-specific educator's guide with sample lesson plans and suggested activities for teachers and group leaders to borrow.

DIRECTIONS

To reach the Route 29 Trailhead, from Interstate 87 take Exit 14 and head west on Union Avenue toward Saratoga Springs. At the first traffic light, turn right onto Henning Road. At the intersection with Lake Avenue/Route 29 (another light), make a right. Go through the traffic light at Weibel Avenue. The trail and parking area is about 300 yards on your right.

Contact: Saratoga P.L.A.N.
112 Spring Street
Saratoga Springs, NY 12866
(518) 587-5554
www.saratogaplan.org/trail_bogmeadow.html

Catskill Scenic Trail

T he Catskill Scenic Trail lives up to its name as it winds through a broad farming valley and small towns in New York's Catskill Mountains. The West Branch of the Delaware River is often in sight with opportunities for fishing and wading in the river's cool waters. The route is primarily agricultural and can at times take your breath away, especially when the farm fields have recently been fertilized.

The trail's west end is in the village of Bloomville. A short path downhill from the parking lot on Agway Road takes you across Route 10 and to the rail-trail. The Sheffield Farm Dairy plant located in Bloomfield contained the country's first milk pasteurization facility. The Ulster and Delaware railroad trains served the plant in the early 1900s. Some restoration work is currently underway on the dilapidated building. Continuing east, a series of bridges carry the trail back and forth across the river, and fishing access points are numerous.

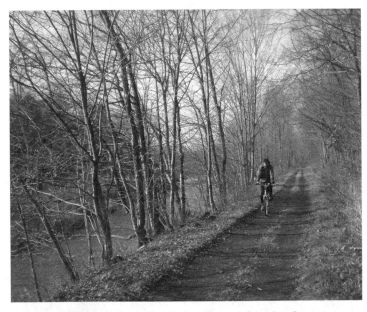

The Catskill Scenic Trail winds through a broad farming valley and small towns in New York.

Location
Delaware and
Schoharie counties

Endpoints
Bloomville to
Roxbury

Mileage
26

**Roughness
Index**
2

Surface
Cinder, dirt and
crushed stone

57

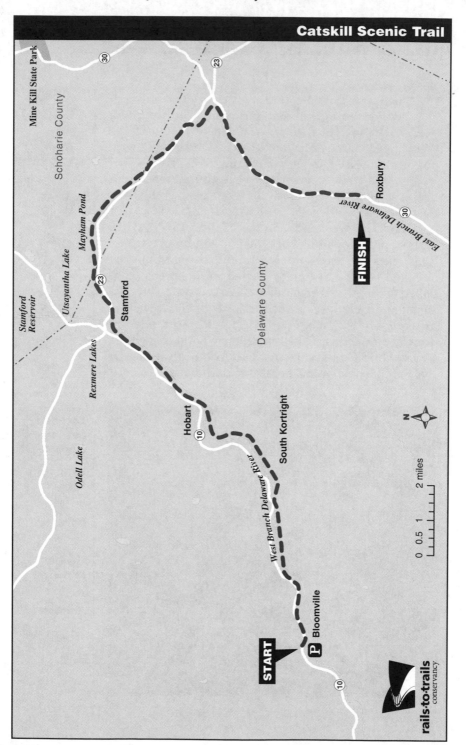

Catskill Scenic Trail

In South Kortright the trail passes through a farmyard. Be prepared—and use caution—when resident turkeys approach looking for a handout. After crossing Route 10 again you will pass the beautiful Belle Terre facility. Formally a private estate, the grounds now house a substance abuse rehabilitation center.

The West Branch of the Delaware River runs right along the trail for most of the 4 miles between Hobart and Stamford. There are some pretty spots to relax with a book or enjoy a picnic; consider heading in to Hobart via Maple Street to stock up on refreshments or to browse the used bookstores on Main Street.

Entering Stamford the restored train station serves as an information center and houses the Catskill Revitalization Corporation, which owns and manages the Catskill Scenic Trail as well as the nearby Delaware and Ulster scenic railroad. Stamford sits at the base of 3,241-foot Mount Utsayantha. The mountain is named for a local American Indian legend and the tragic maiden at the heart of the story.

For the last 5 miles from Stamford to Grand Gorge, the trail remains near the river, and here you can see signs of busy beavers creating dams, building lodges, and occasionally dropping a tree across the trail.

The trail continues on for another 7 miles to the village of Roxbury. Most of this segment of the trail follows the banks of the East Branch of the Delaware River, passing many interesting rock formations.

DIRECTIONS

To reach Bloomville, from Interstate 88 in Oneonta take the exit for State Route 28 toward Delhi for 20.7 miles. Turn left on State Route 10 for 7.7 miles. East of the village of Bloomville, look for Agway Road (also know as Feed Store Road) on the left.

To reach Roxbury, from Interstate 87 take the exit for New York State Route 23 West. In Grand Gorge, turn south on New York State Route 30. The trail begins at Hard Scrabble Road. There is limited parking along the shoulder of the road.

Contact: Catskill Revitalization Corporation
P.O. Box 310
Stamford, NY 12167
(607) 652-2821
http://catskillscenictrail.org

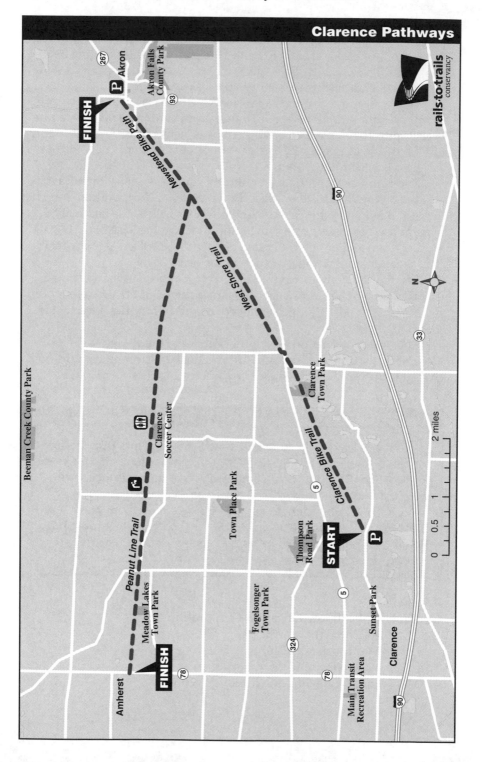

Clarence Pathways

Clarence Pathways: West Shore Trail, Newstead Bike Path, Peanut Line Trail, and Clarence Bike Trail

Four trails make up the Clarence Pathways trail system: the 3.5-mile West Shore Trail, 4.8-mile Newstead Bike Path, 6.1-mile Clarence Bike Trail and 2.3-mile Peanut Line Trail. The trails radiate around the Buffalo suburbs of Clarence, Akron and Amherst.

The 3.5-mile West Shore Trail in Clarence follows the West Shore & Buffalo Railroad corridor. This same corridor saw the very first passenger train stop in Clarence, enroute to Buffalo from Syracuse, on January 1, 1884. The asphalt-paved West Shore Trail travels the rural outskirts of Clarence and connects a number of the town's parks with residential areas and the downtown. Traveling east the trail is bookended by rural farms and fields. In Clarence Town Park the trail shares a low-volume local road for 0.8 mile that provides access to the park and the park maintenance facility.

As the trail passes through downtown Clarence, bike route signs keep you on track. Look for bike lanes on the sidewalk and brick pavers at street crossings. The West Shore Trail returns to a rural setting until reaching Davidson Road. Here the trail becomes the Newstead Bike Path, though there is little noticeable difference between the two.

After 2.5 miles of passing through farmland and woodlots on the Newstead Bike Path, you reach Akron Junction and the connection to the Peanut Line Trail. The Newstead Bike Path continues north and east for another 2 miles through country landscape and near residential developments to the town of Akron.

If you choose to branch off on the Peanut Line Trail you will follow a 6-mile rail-trail that stretches west toward East Amherst. The trail is named for the New York Central Railroad corridor it travels, dubbed the "Peanut Line" for its short length. The first 2.3 miles of the trail, in Newstead, are primarily rural farmland.

When you reach the Newstead-Clarence town line, the Peanut Line Trail becomes the Clarence Bike Trail, though it is also known as the Peanut Line Trail. The Clarence Bike Trail continues west for another 6.1 miles

Location
Erie County

Endpoints
Clarence to Akron

Mileage
16.7

Roughness Index
1

Surface
Asphalt

61

on the old rail line. The trail ends near Transit Road, but not before whisking you through Clarence, where the surroundings gradually become more suburban and residential. Farm fields give way to front yards and, at about 2.4 miles, the trail connects with a community park. A number of side paths snake toward the trail, linking neighborhoods to the popular path.

A walk or a bike ride on any one of the trails within the Clarence Pathways system makes for a delightful outing. Combined, they add up to a daylong adventure.

DIRECTIONS

To reach the trailhead for the West Shore Trail, from State Route 5, turn onto Gunnville Road. Turn right onto Wehrle Drive. The trailhead will be on your right. There is a large parking lot.

To reach the Newstead Bike Path, from State Route 5, take State Route 93 north toward Akron. Stay on Route 93 through Akron. The path ends at the intersection of Cedar (Route 93), Railroad and Eckerson Streets. There is limited curbside parking at this location.

To reach the west end of the Clarence Bike Trail, from State Route 5, take State Route 78 north. The trail endpoint is just north of Muegel Road on the right (east) side of Route 78. There is no public parking at this location.

Contact: Town of Clarence
One Town Place
Clarence, NY 14031
(716) 741-8930
www.erie.gov/clarence

D & H Canal Heritage Corridor

Sandwiched between the Hudson River and the Catskill Mountains near the busy US Route 209 corridor, this trail has a little something for everyone. The Delaware & Hudson Canal Heritage Corridor (D & H Canal), which contains the Ontario and Western Rail-Trail (O & W Rail-Trail), has a southern end with a natural surface that welcomes equestrians, walkers, mountain bikers and winter sports enthusiasts. The northern 2 miles adjacent to US 209 are asphalt paved and add inline skaters, road bikers and wheelchair users to the mix.

The D & H Canal was built in the 1820s to bring coal from the mountains of Pennsylvania to New York City markets. Laborers used picks and shovels to dig the 108-mile system. The canal operated until 1898 when it made the transition to faster and year-round rail transportation.

Entering the trail from the south, off Rest Plaus Road in Marbletown, you are surrounded by a dense forest of primarily deciduous trees native to the area. Farmland is occasionally visible through the wood line.

The hamlet of High Falls, at approximately mile 2, provides intriguing off-trail diversions. The D & H Canal Museum is just a block east from where the trail

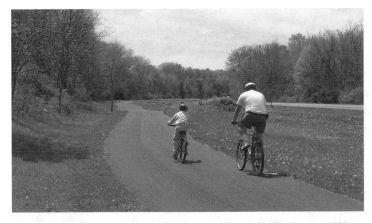

The northern 2 miles adjacent to US 209 are paved to include inline skaters, road bikers and wheelchair users.

Location
Ulster County

Endpoints
Marbletown to Kingston

Mileage
10.4

Roughness Index
2

Surface
Asphalt, dirt and crushed stone

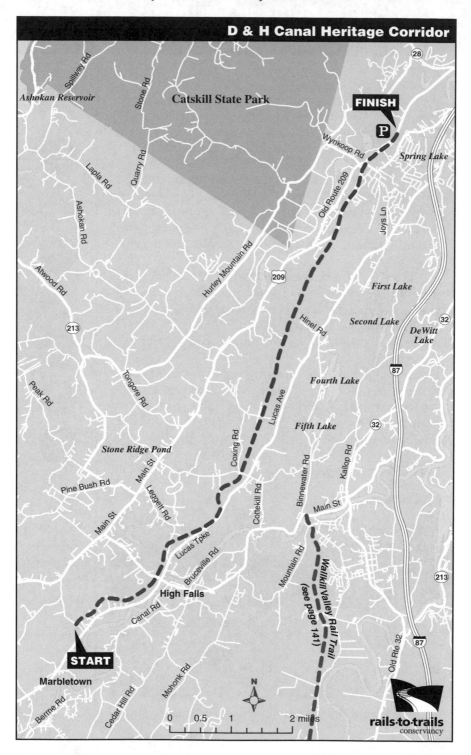

D & H Canal Heritage Corridor

Ashokan Reservoir

Catskill State Park

FINISH

P

Spring Lake

Wynkoop Rd

Spillway Rd

Stone Rd

Quarry Rd

Lapla Rd

Ashokan Rd

Old Route 209

Joys Ln

Atwood Rd

Hurley Mountain Rd

209

First Lake

213

Hinel Rd

Second Lake

DeWitt Lake

32

87

Peak Rd

Tongore Rd

Lucas Ave

Fourth Lake

32

Stone Ridge Pond

Coxing Rd

Fifth Lake

Kallop Rd

Pine Bush Rd

Main St

Cottekill Rd

Binnewater Rd

Main St

Leggett Rd

Lucas Tpke

Bruceville Rd

Mountain Rd

Wallkill Valley Rail Trail
(see page 141)

213

High Falls

Canal Rd

START

87

Old Rte 32

Marbletown

Berme Rd

Cedar Hill Rd

Mohonk Rd

N

0   0.5   1   2 miles

rails·to·trails
conservancy

crosses State Route 213. There are also interesting shops and restaurants. Art galleries, antique shops, cafes and B&Bs can be found along the village's tree-lined streets.

The trail stretches through more wooded terrain with occasional glimpses of the Catskill Mountains to the west. Reaching US Route 209, the trail turns to run parallel to the roadway and is paved for 2.1 miles. Landscaping (trees and shrubs separating the trail from the busy highway) is sponsored and maintained by area businesses and civic organizations. Eagle Scouts have constructed kiosks and benches along this section of the trail.

The D & H Canal Corridor Heritage Alliance, a nonprofit organization dedicated to preserving the Delaware & Hudson Canal towpaths and the Ontario & Western Railway for recreation, is working to open additional miles of this historic pathway.

DIRECTIONS

To reach Marbletown, from US Route 209, turn onto Old Kings Highway. At a fork in the road proceed straight onto Rest Plaus Road. This location *doesn't* have parking.

To reach the trailhead in Kingston, proceed south on US Route 209. Just after crossing the bridge over Esopus Creek, you will see trailhead parking on the left.

Contact: D & H Heritage Corridor Alliance
P.O. Box 176
Rosendale, NY 12472
(845) 647-5292
www.dandhcorridor.org

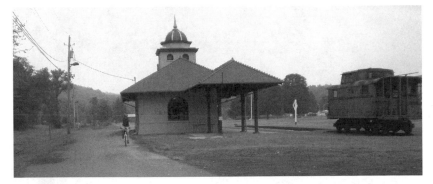

The D & H Canal Museum is just a block east from where the trail crosses State Route 213.

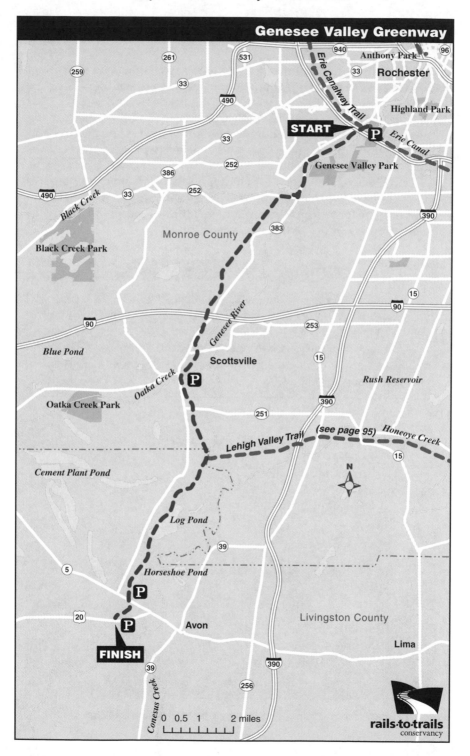

Genesee Valley Greenway

940 Anthony Park 96
261 531
259 33 Rochester
33
490 Highland Park
33
START P Erie Canal
252 Genesee Valley Park
386
252 383
490 33 Monroe County
Black Creek
Black Creek Park 390
15
90 90
253
Blue Pond Genesee River
Scottsville 15
P Rush Reservoir
Oatka Creek
Oatka Creek Park 390
251
Lehigh Valley Trail (see page 95) Honeoye Creek
Cement Plant Pond 15
N
Log Pond
39
5 Horseshoe Pond
P
20 Avon Livingston County
P Lima
FINISH
39 390
256

Conesus Creek
0 0.5 1 2 miles

rails·to·trails
conservancy

Genesee Valley Greenway

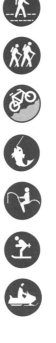

The Genesee Valley Greenway is a 90-mile ribbon of open space, rolling through towns and countless landscapes from Rochester to Cuba, New York. The greenway is a work in progress, but the 18 miles from Rochester south to Avon provide a continuous off-road trail experience. Some open sections south of Avon require on-road riding to make the connections and other sections that are unimproved with bridges missing. The greenway follows the old transportation routes of the Genesee Valley Canal and the Rochester Branch of the Pennsylvania Railroad. Historic villages, connections with other trails, and relics such as surviving canal structures provide a rich layer to this otherwise rural ride.

Only the first 2 miles of the Greenway are paved. Cinder, grass and packed dirt give the rest of the trail a firm, level platform.

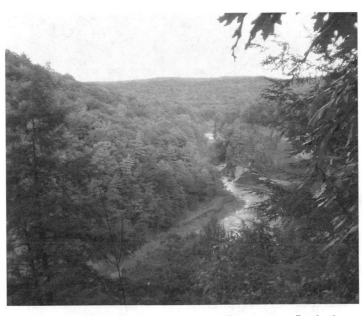

The greenway may be a work in progress, but it provides a continuous off-road trail experience from Rochester to Avon.

Location
Monroe and
Livingston counties

Endpoints
Rochester to Avon

Mileage
18

Roughness Index
2

Surface
Asphalt, cinder, dirt and grass

67

From the start at Rochester's Genesee Valley Park are intriguing sights: You pass the Rochester International Airport fire training school and two charred airplane fuselages used in demonstrations. A short on-road detour along State Route 383 and Ballantyne Road takes you off and then back to the trail. A short side trail takes you north over historic Black Creek Culvert (circa 1838), one of the state's largest 19th-century canal culverts, before it dead-ends at an active rail corridor.

Back on the greenway you pass a large tract of forest conserved by the Genesee Land Trust. At mile 5.5 is the impressive stone Canal Lock #2, one of the few surviving locks along the Greenway.

The village of Scottsville, at mile 9, has connected itself to the trail via the Canal Street Boardwalk. After a detour into the village for refreshments, you can head across Oatka Creek to Canawaugus Park, with picnic tables, parking and a view across the creek to some remaining historic canal structures. Portions of the old canal bed have become a wetland habitat. Over the next several miles wildlife abounds, attracting bird watchers and nature photographers.

In Wadsworth Junction, at mile 12.5, you can see massive stone abutments from the bridge that carried the Lehigh Valley Railroad across the Pennsylvania Railroad route. Today both rail corridors are parks. The Lehigh Valley Trail (see page 95) travels 15 miles east across Monroe County. In the trail's first few hundred feet, a short distance

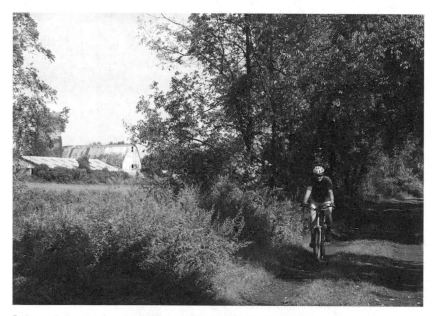

Farther south, the views from the greenway are primarily rural and agricultural.

east, users are carried over the Genesee River on the same railroad bridge that carried Lehigh Valley cars on its upper deck.

Continuing south, the views from the greenway are primarily rural and agricultural. Occasional wood stands interrupt the otherwise expansive farming landscape. Horses and cattle graze in pastures. Farmhouses, barns and other outbuildings punctuate vast swaths of soybeans, corn and cabbage.

South of Avon, the Genesee Valley Greenway is a work in progress. Sections have been improved, but some bridges are missing, and other sections detour onto the road. Friends of the Genesee Valley Greenway's website (www.fogvg.org) contains a detailed map and a mile-by-mile trail description.

DIRECTIONS

To reach Rochester, from Interstate 390 in Rochester, exit onto Scottsville Road/State Route 383. Turn left onto Scottsville Road. At the first traffic light, turn right onto Genesee Park Boulevard. At the T intersection turn right again. There is a large parking lot on the left near the tennis courts. At the rear of the parking lot, you will find the Canalway Trail. Follow this trail to the west (don't cross the bridge) to the start of the Genesee Valley Greenway.

There is a large parking area for trail users on the north side of US Route 20 (Telephone Road) to the west of the village of Avon. From Avon, take US Route 20/State Route 5 west. Stay on US 20/ Telephone Road. There is a large parking lot on the north side of US 20 before the intersection with River Road.

Contact: Friends of the Genesee Valley Greenway
P.O. Box 42
Mt. Morris, NY 14510
(585) 658-2569
www.fogvg.org

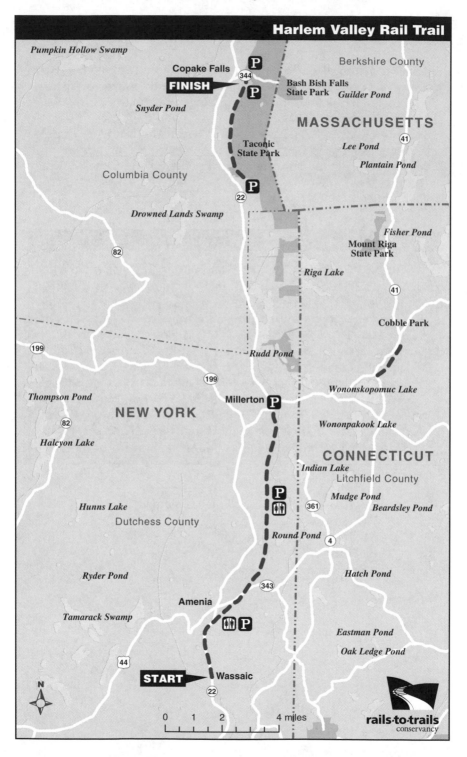

Harlem Valley Rail Trail

The Harlem Valley Rail Trail provides a scenic ride through rolling farm fields and dense woods on the bed of the New York and Harlem Railroad that ran from New York City to Chatham, New York. The rail-trail has been built in segments, and there is still work to be done to open all 46 miles of the planned trail. For now you can take in two segments, which total 15 miles, and get a good sense of how sweet the future is for this rail-trail.

The southern end of the trail begins at the Metro North Railroad Station in Wassaic, New York. It is possible, during non-rush hours and on weekends, to board a Metro North train in Grand Central Station and in a little more than two hours be peddling or walking along this rail-trail. As the trail points north for nearly 11 miles to Millerton, it passes through a pastoral scene. Farmland stretches before and around you, followed by red cedar scrubland and beaver ponds. In Amenia, the

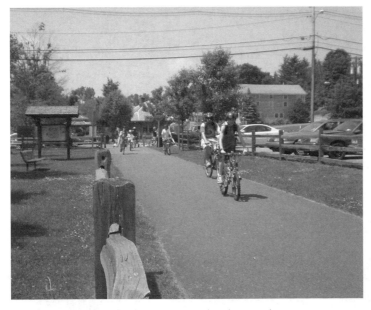

As the trail heads north to Millerton, it passes through a pastoral scene.

Location
Dutchess and Columbia counties

Endpoints
Metro North Railroad Station in Wassaic to Taconic State Park in Copake Falls

Mileage
14.8

Roughness Index
1

Surface
Asphalt

71

trailhead parking lot is on the site of the former Barton House, a large hotel that was frequented by business people and vacationers traveling from New York City.

Several railroad stations on this line have been restored: Sharon Station is now a private residence located off the trail in the town of North East. Millerton's three stations have been restored and today house local businesses. North of Coleman Station the trail crosses six reconstructed railroad bridges.

The railroad builders tamed the area's rolling terrain, and created a level corridor, by blasting through rock and building the rail bed up from the land adjacent to the corridor for a "pyramiding" effect. In several stretches, north of Route 61, the trail's higher elevation on steep embankments—in some places dropping 50 feet—provides spectacular views of the surrounding farmland. Indian Mountain, straddling the border of New York and Connecticut, is to the east. Traveling through a series of deep rock cuts, you will feel the temperature drop several degrees from the surrounding landscape.

Millerton is the current end of the first section of rail-trail. In Millerton, two restored train stations that appear to have changed little since their original construction in 1851 and 1912, respectively, flank the trail. A third station, once used for freight, stands nearby. All house local businesses today. The village offers ample opportunities for refreshment and shopping.

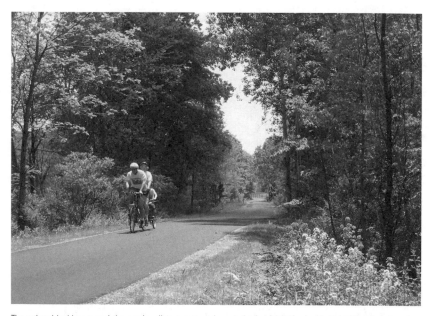

The railroad builders tamed the area's rolling terrain and created a level corridor by blasting through rock and building the rail bed up from the adjacent land.

The next 8 miles of the railroad corridor between Main Street in Millerton and Under Mountain Road in Ancram are not open for public use.

Reaching the next open trail section requires a detour on a two-lane road. Head west on Main Street in Millerton, and then north on New York State Route 22 for about 7.7 miles. Turn right on Under Mountain Road and look for the trailhead on the left. The 4-mile paved section of trail between Under Mountain Road and Taconic State Park is more wooded as the trail hugs the base of the South Taconic Mountains.

About 2.9 miles north of Under Mountain Road, the trail detours onto a scenic dirt road for 0.4 mile to bypass a privately held parcel of rail bed. The dirt road rejoins the paved rail-trail for another half mile to the entrance to Taconic State Park at Copake Falls. Scenic Bash Bish Falls are located about a mile east of the trailhead, just over the Massachusetts state border. Follow the hiking trail to reach the falls.

DIRECTIONS

To reach the Wassaic trailhead, from Interstate 84 or Interstate 684, take State Route 22 north at Brewster. Continue north on Route 22 to the Wassaic Station of the Metro North Railroad. The station is on the right side of the road.

To reach the Taconic State Park Trailhead, from Interstate 84 or Interstate 684, take State Route 22 north to Brewster. Continue north on Route 22 to State Route 344, about 6 miles north of Millerton. Turn right and proceed about a half mile to the triangular green. Bear to the left to the stop sign. Proceed straight about a third of a mile to the entrance of Taconic State Park; ask the attendant where to park.

Contact: Harlem Valley Rail Trail Association, Inc.
51 South Center St.
P.O. Box 356
Millerton, NY 12546
(518) 789-9591
www.hvrt.org

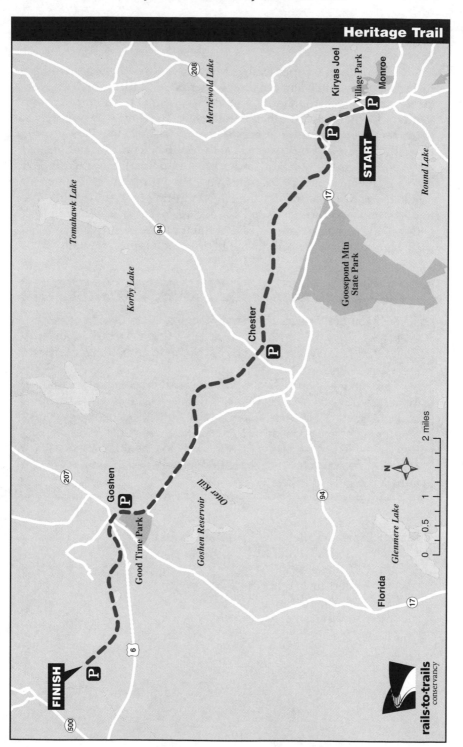

Heritage Trail

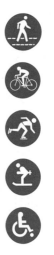

Much of the trail, also known as the Orange Heritage Trail, sails past wide fields of corn and wheat. The right-of-way is 11.5 miles, but a gap in the west end creates two distinct trails, a 9.1-mile paved section and a 2.4-mile unpaved segment. With the exception of the half-mile on-road detour in between, there are only a few street crossings, making this an ideal destination for families with young children.

The longer portion of the Heritage Trail starts in Monroe at Crane Park, also called Airplane Park for the old Saber fighter jet in a corner of the park along Mill Pond Parkway. The smooth pavement here draws bicyclists, inline skaters, wheelchair users and parents with strollers. Just beyond the park Orange-Rockland Lake dominates the view to the right.

The park and ride lot along Orange and Rockland Road makes the trail an excellent active transportation corridor for commuters taking public transit.

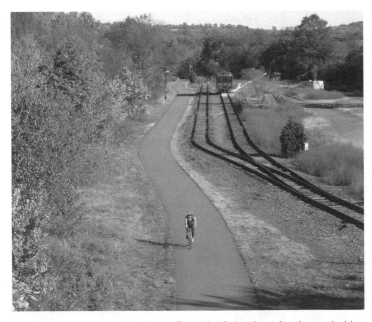

The smooth pavement of the Heritage Trail is ideal for bicyclists, inline skaters, wheelchair users and parents with strollers.

Location
Orange County

Endpoints
Hartley Road in Goshen to Airplane Park in Monroe

Mileage
11.5

Roughness Index
1

Surface
Asphalt and crushed stone

75

In the village of Chester is a unique stone façade restored train station that serves as the Chester Depot Museum. Shops in the village offer mid-trip refreshments. Before you reach the village, you pass an old cemetery with weathered headstones dating to the 1800s. Between Chester and Goshen, the trail is lined with trees as it passes through farmland and wood lots and past residential developments.

The road detour begins with the end of the trail's paved section at St. James Place in Goshen. The traffic control signals and crosswalks make the detour easy to follow. Follow the long narrow parking lot for two blocks, crossing Bruen Place and Greenwich Avenue. After crossing Greenwich Avenue, proceed as straight as possible to cross West Maine Street using the well-marked pedestrian crosswalk. Cross Grand Street using the pedestrian crosswalk and proceed on the sidewalk to cross Grant Street. Proceed around the right side of the restored railroad depot that now serves as the Goshen police station. Follow Railroad Avenue around a townhouse development to connect to the remaining 2.4 miles of unpaved trail

These 2.4 miles of trail are like a quiet country cousin of the paved section to the east. Other than passing under Route 17 you won't see a lot of other development. You will see birders and equestrians enjoying this less well-developed trail's rural surroundings. This section currently ends at Hartley Road but will be extended toward Middletown in the future.

DIRECTIONS

To reach Airplane Park (also known as Crane Park) in Monroe, take Exit 130 off Route 17 onto Route 208 to Monroe. Bear right at the fork to a traffic light. Turn left at the light and make the first left onto Mill Pond Parkway. The park is on the left.

To reach the Goshen Trailhead, from Interstate 84, take Exit 3 onto US Route 6 and State Route 17M heading east. Turn left onto Hartley Road. The beginning of the trail is on the left. There is limited parking at this location.

Contact: Orange County Department of Parks and Recreation
211 Route 416
Montgomery, NY 12549
(845) 457-4900
www.co.orange.ny.us

High Line

S tart spreading the news about New York City's innovative new public park. The High Line rail-trail is an urban marvel, stretching 1.5 miles and towering almost 30 feet above street level through several neighborhoods in the lower west side of Manhattan. The first section of the High Line was opened in 2009 and runs approximately 10 blocks from Gansevoort Street to the north entrance at 20th Street.

The corridor was built in the 1930s to remove rail traffic from streets bustling with industry. The elevated design improved street-level safety and allowed freight cars to roll directly into the buildings so that workers could load livestock and meats at the slaughterhouses and agricultural goods at factories and warehouses. The corridor fell into disuse in 1980. While owners of property under the High Line lobbied—unsuccessfully—to level the structure and make way for development, the neglected corridor quietly turned into an overgrown natural landscape.

Location
New York City

Endpoints
Gansevoort Street
to 20th Street

Mileage
0.7

Roughness Index
1

Surface
Concrete

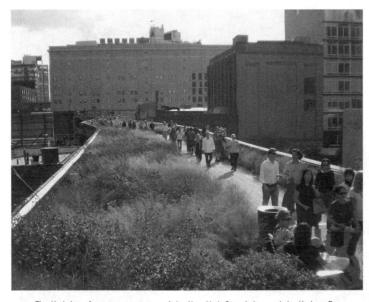

The High Line features a rare view of the New York City skyline and the Hudson River with the amenities of a popular public park.

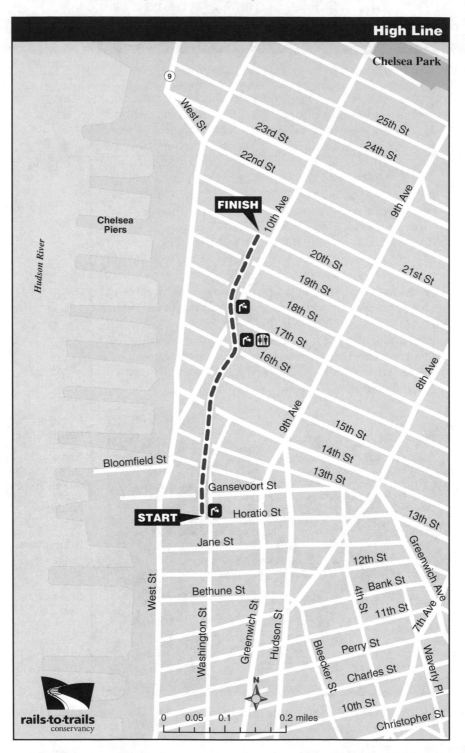

In 1999 Chelsea residents Joshua David and Robert Hammond founded an organization to preserve the demolition-bound corridor as a public park. Friends of the High Line waged a hard-won battle that resulted in the support of city officials and, in 2005, the transfer of High Line ownership from the CSX rail company to New York City.

To experience the High Line is to have a rare view of the city skyline and the Hudson River, with the amenities (and restrictions) of a popular public park. The finished portion of the greenway artfully incorporates characteristics of the old corridor. Sections of original railroad track are visible in the concrete slab designs that make up the surface of the path. Other sections of the trail reveal original art-deco steel railings paired with modern wooden benches that organically connect to the concrete surface.

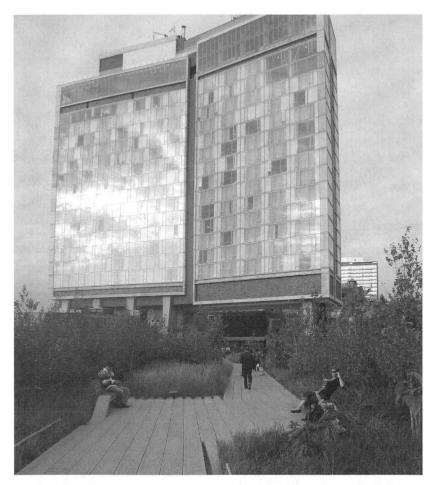

Covering 1.5 miles, the High Line towers almost 30 feet above street level and winds through several neighborhoods on the lower west side of Manhattan.

Heading north from Gansevoort Street in the Meatpacking District, you pass through a series of unique features, including the Gansevoort Wodland, Washington Grasslands, Sun Decks and Water Features, Chelsea Grasslands 23rd Street Lawn and a Wildflower Field. The grasslands and gardens have been planted with many of the wild grasses and other self-seeding plants found on the corridor during the 25 years it lay dormant. The overall effect is a wholesome combination of organic beauty and stylized form that will leave you longing for more. Here is the good news: The second section of the High Line from 20th Street to 30th Street is scheduled to open in 2011.

DIRECTIONS

The trail is open daily from 7 A.M. to 10 P.M. (8 P.M. in winter). There are access points at Gansevoort Street, 14th, 16th, 18th and 20th streets. Elevators are located at 14th and 16th streets. When the park reaches peak capacity during the summer season, you may be required to access the High Line from Gansevoort Street. Bicycling is prohibited, but bike racks are located on street-level at most access points.

The Gansevoort Street entrance can be reached via several methods of public transportation, including the A / C / E / L to 14th Street and 8th Avenue, 1 / 2 / 3 to 14th Street and 7th Avenue, M11 to Hudson and West 14th streets, M11 to Washington Street, M11 to 9th Avenue and M14 to 9th Avenue.

The 20th Street entrance can be reached via several methods of public transportation, including C / E to 23rd Street and 8th Avenue, 1 to 23rd Street and 7th Avenue, M23 to 10th Avenue and M34 to 10th Avenue.

Contact: Friends of the High Line
529 West 20th Street, Suite 8W
New York, NY 10011
(202) 206-9922
www.thehighline.org

Hojack Trail

This pleasant community trail connects suburban residences close to the shore of Lake Ontario with a school, a church and a commercial area in Webster, New York. Near the trail's northwest end, it connects with old-growth forests and unique coastal lands preserved by the town.

The trail takes its name from the Lake Ontario Shore Railroad's "Hojack Line" that served the area's apple orchards and other agriculturally based businesses. The tread varies from small sections of crushed stone to packed cinder ballast and mowed grass.

Starting at the trailhead at Vosburg Hollow Nature Preserve gives you instant access to a wooded hilltop hiking path, the Vosburg Hollow Nature Trail, which leads you about an eighth of a mile through a red pine forest to the longer Vosburg Hiking Trail and the Gosnell Big Woods Preserve beyond. The branch trail offers

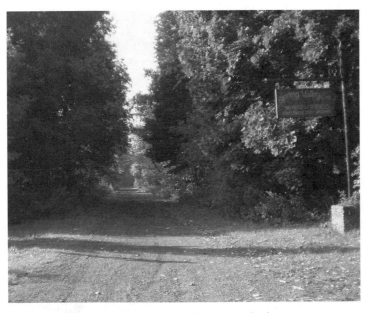

The Hojack Trail passes through sections of deciduous wood and grasses.

Location
Cayuga County

Endpoints
Lake Road to Holt
Road in Webster

Mileage
3.5

**Roughness
Index**
3

Surface
Cinder and dirt

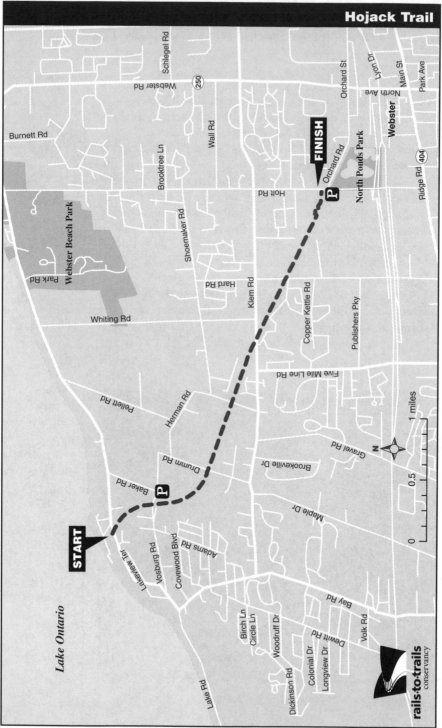

Hojack Trail

a bike rack so you can lock up your bike and continue on foot to the top of the hill.

Staying on the Hojack rail-trail, you can head less than a half mile north and west of the trailhead to Lake Road. You cannot, however, reach the shore or get a good vista point until you travel west on Lake Road for a quarter mile.

Heading east the rail-trail passes through sections of deciduous wood and grasses. The route looks and feels remote, but is never very far from busy roads and homes. It is only when you come to the half-dozen road crossings that you realize you are not, in fact, traveling through the wilderness.

For now, the trail comes to an abrupt end between Hard and Holt roads. You can exit the trail at Hard Road or opt to continue on foot through a small nature park called North Ponds Park, and make your way out through a condominium complex onto Holt Road. Better yet, head back toward the Vosburg Hollow Nature Trail for a longer adventure.

DIRECTIONS

To reach the trailhead at the Vosburg Hollow Nature Preserve from Route 104, turn north onto Bay Road and continue for 1.5 miles. Make a right on Lake Road. Then in 0.2 mile bear right onto Vosburg Road. Follow Vosburg Road for a half mile. Parking is at the Vosburg Hollow Nature Preserve on the right and behind the water treatment facility.

Contact: Friends of Webster Trails
595 Bending Bough Drive
Webster, NY 14580
www.webstertrails.org

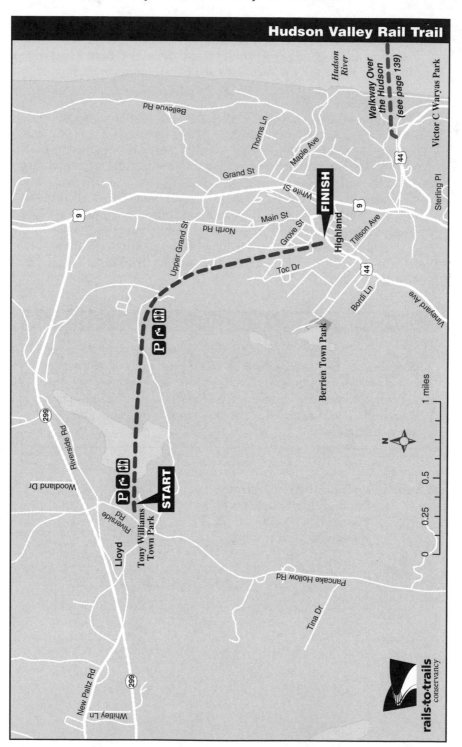

Hudson Valley Rail Trail

Hudson Valley Rail Trail

Located in the mid-Hudson Valley is a remarkable trail that is picturesque and family friendly. This flat, paved trail stretches a little more than 2 miles through hardwood forests, over Black Creek and under two spectacular stone arch bridges. The trail stretches between the towns of Highland and Lloyd on the former right-of-way of the New York, New Haven and Hartford Railroad. Ulster County acquired the line when the railroad went bankrupt, and the county deeded the section from the Hudson River to Route 299 to the town of Lloyd.

The corridor sat vacant until the town sold an easement for the installation of a fiber optic cable along the unused line. With funding in place, the citizens of Lloyd and members of the Highland Rotary Club prepared for trail development by clearing the right-of-way of brush and debris. Some of the old railroad signal structures were left to provide a link to the corridor's past. In 1997 the first section of trail was opened.

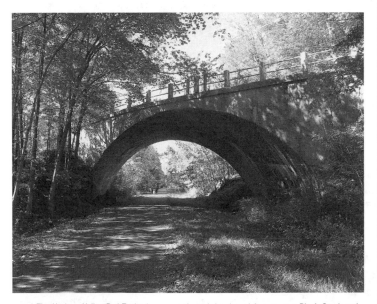

The Hudson Valley Rail Trail takes users through hardwood forests, over Black Creek and under two spectacular stone arch bridges.

Location
Ulster County

Endpoints
Tony Williams Park (Riverside Road off Route 299) in Lloyd to Vineyard Avenue in Highland

Mileage
2.4

Roughness Index
1

Surface
Asphalt

85

From Tony Williams Park in Lloyd the trail heads east though a wooded canopy. Less than a half mile from the park, the trail crosses over Black Creek, which is a popular spot with kayakers and canoeists. Close to mile 1, the trail runs along a rock cut. In the spring, graceful columbine plants sprout out of the cracks in the rock. The cut provides a cool spot to stop and relax on hot summer days.

At the trail's midpoint two magnificent arched bridges carry New Paltz Road over the corridor. Next up is the Highland Rotary Pavilion. The Highland Rotary Club has made the Hudson Valley Rail Trail a primary project for more than a decade. The pavilion has restroom facilities, a large parking lot, a fully restored caboose, picnic tables and water.

As you move east and south, trailside exercise stations let you test your endurance and strength. You are nearing the hamlet of Highland with residential neighborhoods on a less heavily wooded trail.

At the end of the developed portion of the trail lays the promise of the future. A new section of trail extends the Hudson Valley Rail Trail 1.2 miles to the Poughkeepsie-Highland Railroad Bridge. A brand new pedestrian walkway on the old truss bridge, called Walkway Over the Hudson (see page 139), is drawing scores of visitors who want to drink in the view from the milelong, 212-foot-high span across the Hudson River.

DIRECTIONS

To reach the Tony Williams Park in Lloyd, from the New York State Thruway take Exit 18 for Poughkeepsie and New Paltz). At the traffic light at the end of the exit, turn right onto State Route 299 East and go 2.3 miles. Turn right onto New Paltz Road and go 0.7 mile. Turn left onto South Riverside Road; after 0.1 mile turn right into Tony Williams Park. Parking is to the left by the start of the rail-trail.

To reach the Highland Rotary Pavilion in Highland, take State Route 9W to State Route 299 West toward New Paltz. Turn left onto South Chodikee Lake Road. At the end of Chodikee Lake Road, turn right onto New Paltz Road. The parking area for the pavilion is on the left.

Contact: Hudson Valley Rail Trail Association, Inc.
12 Church Street
Highland, NY 12528
(845) 691-2066
http://hudsonvalleyrailtrail.net

Jim Schug Trail

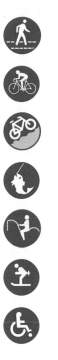

The Jim Schug Trail offers a short, sweet excursion in New York's Finger Lakes region. The trail was known as the Dryden Lake Trail until it was re-named, in 2002, in memory of the late town supervisor who acquired the land. The trail follows a remarkably level Lehigh Valley Railroad corridor; the railroad con-structed the bed by creating cuts and using the removed earth and rock to fill in low spots. The resulting trail is level while the surrounding landscape dips and rises, leaving you on an elevated berm or passing through cuts where ground level is above your head.

There are numerous road crossings—many with small parking areas—that provide easy trail access. From the village of Dryden, the trail runs south and east and, when complete to Harford, it will intersect with the Finger Lakes Trail, a footpath for hikers. Begin on West Main Street at the signboard for the Agway store. A half mile south a railroad bridge carries the trail over Virgil Creek. Benches mark your distance every half mile, and accompanying informational signs reveal historical and natural features along the trail.

When the trail crosses State Route 38, the landscape becomes more rural. Farm fields and silos, woods and wetlands lie ahead. Don't hurry through the next mile but rather sit and listen to the sounds of the wetlands. In the evening, especially in spring, the sounds of frogs surround you.

The area around Dryden Lake and along the trail is said to have some of the best birding in the Finger Lakes region. Dryden Lake Park surrounds the lake and has picnic tables, a pavilion, and fishing access, including a handicapped-accessible platform. All seasons see activ-ity on the lake: Birders flock to the area for waterfowl in the spring and fall. In the winter, the lake is a popular spot for ice fishing.

Adding to the bucolic appeal is an array of cultivat-ed, alien and native plant species. Wildflowers bloom along the trail from spring through autumn, and the

Location
Cortland and Tompkins counties

Endpoints
Dryden to Harford

Mileage
4.2

Roughness Index
2

Surface
Grass and gravel

87

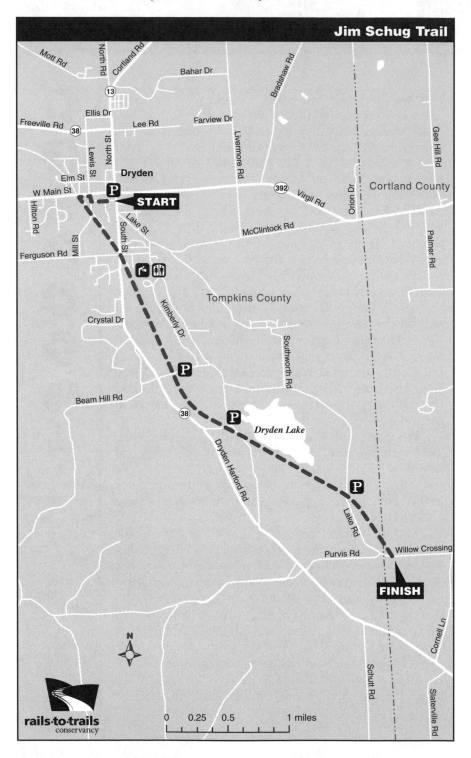

Jim Schug Trail

woods show spectacular fall color. The ever-changing natural palette warrants return visits to this trail throughout the year.

DIRECTIONS

If driving and parking, to reach the Dryden trailhead, you have to pass it first to park. From Ithaca follow Route 13 (Dryden Road), which becomes Main Street. Turn south on Mill Street shortly before the first traffic light in Dryden. Turn left immediately onto George Street. A municipal parking lot is on the right. To reach the trail from the parking lot, retrace your route. Turn right onto George Street and follow it to Mill Street. Turn right onto Mill Street and turn left onto West Main Street. The trail entrance is on the left, opposite Rochester Street and between Don Mayes Photography and Dryden Agway.

Dryden Lake Park offers the most parking opportunities. From downtown Dryden (above), take State Route 38 south for 2 miles and turn left on Chaffee Road into the park. You will cross the trail just before the park entrance.

Contact: Town of Dryden, Department of Public Works
61 East Main Street
Dryden, NY 13053
(607) 884-8654
www.dryden.ny.us/Dryden%20Trails/jim_schug_1.htm

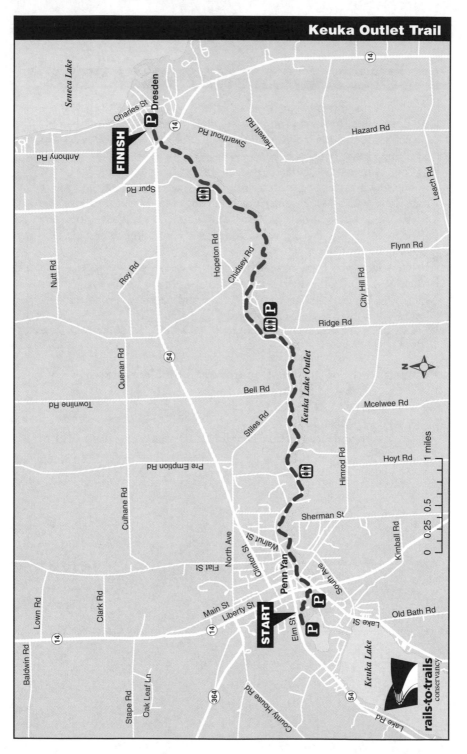

Keuka Outlet Trail

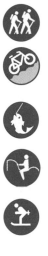

In the heart of New York's Finger Lakes Region is a rail-trail that is part natural wonder and part industrial archaeology. The Keuka Outlet Trail is a unique 7-mile trail with a unique heritage. Technically a stream, the 8-mile Keuka (*KYOO-ka*) Lake Outlet physically connects Keuka Lake to Seneca Lake in the east, the only two Finger Lakes in New York connected by a natural waterway. The outlet also connects the historic lakeside villages of Penn Yan on Keuka Lake (settled in 1833 by Pennsylvania Yankees) and Dresden on Seneca Lake.

Settled in the late 1700s by the Society of Universal Friends, the waterway became a gateway to western New York State. At its height of development in 1830, the 8-mile Keuka Lake Outlet, then called Crooked Lake, supported as many as 40 mills and 12 hydropower dams. The dams powered lumber mills and, to a lesser degree, tanneries, distilleries, and mills producing linseed oil, grain and plaster. As the boon of canal

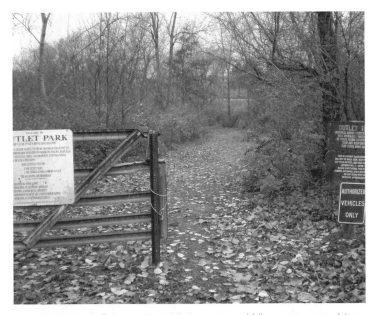

The Keuka Outlet Trail passes through lush vegetation and follows a narrow strip of dirt smoothed by countless bicycle tires.

Location
Yates County

Endpoints
Penn Yan to Dresden

Mileage
7

Roughness Index
3

Surface
Cinder, dirt, gravel and asphalt

91

transportation took hold, New York State built the Crooked Lake Canal along the length of the outlet. It was a colossal venture. Twenty-seven locks were built of stone and wood along the 8-mile waterway (by comparison, the 360-mile Erie Canal has only 90 locks). After an initial positive impact on the economy, the canal required constant repair and construction. The state legislature eventually sold the land, in 1878, to businessmen who converted the canal corridor to the Penn Yan and New York Railroad Company. New York Central ran the railroad until 1972 when floods from Hurricane Agnes destroyed the corridor.

The original canal dropped approximately 270 feet over an 8-mile section between Penn Yan and Dresden to the east. After the locks were removed, a number of waterfalls naturally developed; the waterway now attracts recreational paddlers. The water flow is controlled by a dam at Penn Yan and can change drastically from week to week or even day to day. The trail itself remains fairly level for the entire 7 miles.

The countryside hosts fields of produce farms and vineyards, but remains of mills and dams along the corridor help you feel the ghosts of 19th-century industrial America. Large rusting gears sit silent by beautiful rushing waterfalls; sections of trail meander through remnants of cut stone walls. In most places, the water has reclaimed the land and become a haven for wildlife and waterfowl. It is not unusual to see herons perched at the water's edge.

The majority of the trail passes through lush vegetation and follows a narrow strip of dirt smoothed by countless bicycle tires. Several feet of mowed grass border the dirt path. A short section of trail in Penn Yan is paved with asphalt but the majority of trail is crushed stone and dirt. About the midpoint of the trail, the Seneca Mill Falls picnic area is a popular trailhead and picnic spot near the largest falls along the trail. Approximately 3 miles of the trail from Seneca Mill traveling east to Hopeton Mill cut through a steep gorge carved from shale and limestone during the last ice age. This natural wonder contrasts sharply with the historic mill remnants that trail users can spot periodically at former mill sites along the trail.

The villages of Penn Yan and Dresden are now tourist destinations; the people and businesses are open to sharing the wealth of their heritage with interested visitors. A bike rental is available in Penn Yan and an ice cream shop in Dresden caters to trail users.

DIRECTIONS

To reach the trailhead in Penn Yan, from Main Street, turn west onto Elm Street (Route 54A) and follow to the community ball field on the left. The trail access is behind the vendor booth, to your left, as you are looking at the field.

To reach the Dresden Trailhead, follow Route 54 east to Dresden. After crossing Route 14 bear right onto Seneca Street. The trailhead and parking lot are on the right.

Contact: Friends of the Outlet
P.O. Box 65
Dresden, NY 14441
(315) 536-9484
www.keukaoutlettrail.com

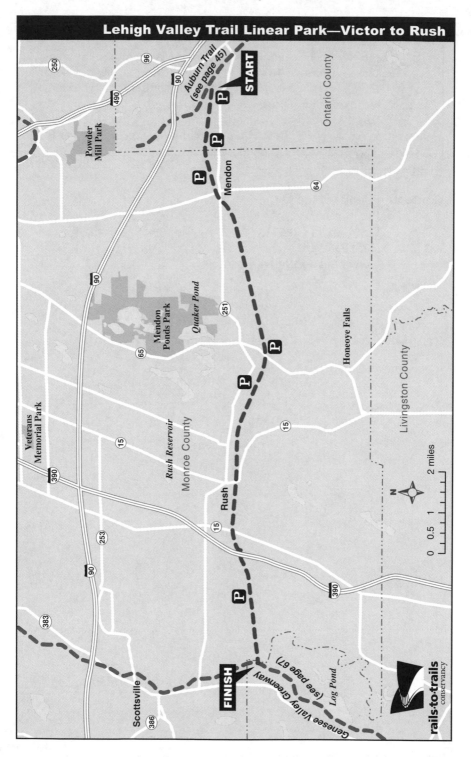

Lehigh Valley Trail Linear Park—Victor to Rush

Lehigh Valley Trail Linear Park– Victor to Rush

The Lehigh Valley Trail is part of a developing system of rail-trails in western New York. The segment from Victor to Rush offers nearly 15 miles of serene wooded and rural areas. Plus, it is literally expanding horizons for trail enthusiasts. The trail connects on the western end with the Genesee Valley Greenway (see page 67) and on the east end to the Auburn Trail (see page 45). About midway the northern extension of Lehigh Valley Trail joins the main segment at Rochester Junction. This developing trail will eventually connect to the Erie Canal Towpath about 5 miles to the north.

Some call this gem of a rail-trail the Black Diamond Trail, which stems from the Lehigh Valley Railroad's nickname, "The Route of the Black Diamond." The railroad's 435-mile main line between Buffalo and New York City was used for hauling anthracite coal (black diamonds) from Pennsylvania.

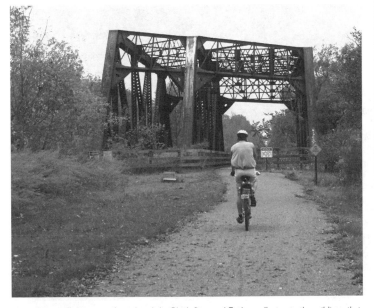

Some call this gem of a rail-trail the Black Diamond Trail, an allusion to the rail lines that ran anthracite coal (black diamonds) through the area.

Location
Monroe and Ontario counties

Endpoints
Victor to Rush

Mileage
14.6

Roughness Index
1

Surface
Crushed stone

95

Start in Victor, where the most convenient parking, at the Phillips Road Trailhead, provides the option to explore the Auburn Trail as well. The Lehigh Valley Trail's newly decked trestle bridge is visible from the parking area; west of the bridge is the short connector to the Auburn Trail.

Heading west, the Lehigh Valley Trail is a smooth crushed stone path. Equestrians are encouraged to preserve the trail surface by using the 5-foot grassy space that parallels the trail.

This is the trail's most recently built section. You have open views of meadows and some industrial park buildings, but trees soon enclose the corridor. Around mile 1 you reach a small park with picnic tables in a pavilion and a section of preserved railroad track. You might want to leave the trail to explore the quaint hamlet of Mendon and pick up a snack.

Beyond the park are the town's athletic fields. As the woods become denser, watch for deer. From this point on the view from the trail alternates between wooded sections and farm fields with occasional horse paddocks. Near the midpoint a kiosk in Rochester Junction tells the history of the railroad spur that ran to Rochester. This is now the 3.5-mile Lehigh Valley Trail Northern Extension that leads, with some on-road sections, to Henrietta. Note a wooden fence outlining the footprint of the original country depot.

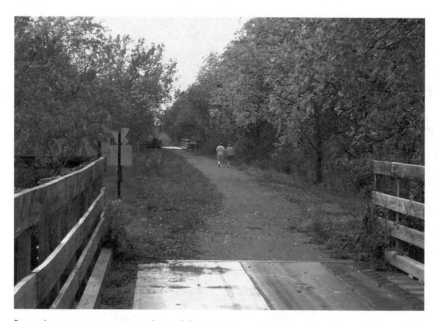

Deer sightings are more common as the woods become denser.

As you approach pretty Honeoye Creek and its forested wetlands keep your eyes open for red-winged blackbirds. At about mile 10.5 in Rush Veterans Memorial Park is a viewing platform above the creek. If you've worked up an appetite, the town of Rush has a few places to eat just off the trail, but don't miss the trail's grand finale. At its western end, before connecting in a T-bone fashion with the Genesee Valley Greenway, an old railroad bridge gives you a grand perspective on the lovely Genesee River.

DIRECTIONS

To reach the Phillips Road Trailhead near Victor, from the New York Thruway (Route 90), take Exit 45 and follow Route 96 South. Turn right on Main Street in Fishers (Route 42), then left on Phillips Road. Go about a mile, watching for a trail crosswalk on the road. The first parking area is for the Auburn Trail; the second is for the Lehigh Valley Trail.

Contact: Town of Victor Parks and Recreation
1290 Blossom Drive
Victor, NY 14564
(585) 924-1840
www.victorny.org

Monroe County Parks
171 Reservoir Avenue
Rochester, NY 14620
(585) 753-PARK (7275)
www.monroecounty.gov

Mohawk-Hudson Bike-Hike Trail

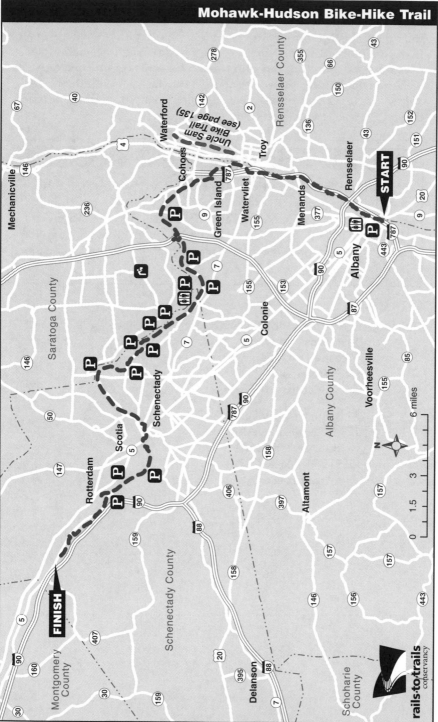

Mohawk-Hudson Bike-Hike Trail

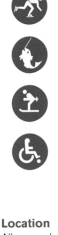

This diverse rail-trail travels through five municipalities, connects ten parks, parallels two rivers and offers dozens of scenic views. It is a mostly continuous asphalt-paved trail with some on-road sections. The trail is the easternmost stretch of the Erie Canalway, which traverses the state from Albany to Buffalo. The Mohawk-Hudson (named for the two rivers it traces) is a 39-mile treat of woods, meadows and rivers interspersed with city and suburban neighborhoods. One of the on-road detours is through Schenectady's well-preserved historical Stockade district.

Built in a piecemeal fashion in the late 1970s and early 80s, this trail is still called by a different name in almost every town. In addition to referring to the map on the facing page, you can get a detailed trail map, as well as a regional bike map, free from the Capital District Transportation Committee.

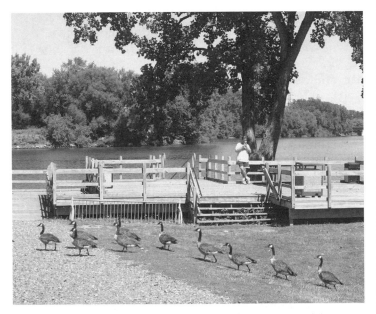

The Mohawk-Hudson Bike-Hike Trail goes through woods and meadows and along rivers, interspersed with city and suburban neighborhoods.

Location
Albany and Schenectady counties

Endpoints
Corning Riverfront Preserve in Albany to Route 5S near Rotterdam Junction

Mileage
39

Roughness Index
1

Surface
Asphalt

A good place to start is Albany's popular Corning Riverfront Preserve, easily accessible from Interstate 787 South and close to the trail's southern end. Head a half mile to the trail's start at Riverfront Amphitheater and Hudson River Way Pedestrian Bridge, where you are rewarded with striking views of downtown Albany. Then turn around and head north with the interstate to your left and the Hudson River on your right. This portion of trail features woods and meadows, opening from time to time to river views.

After passing under I-787 at mile 4.8, you are diverted on city streets for about 4 miles. The bike route is well signed and manageable for cyclists used to riding with traffic. Don't miss the museum at the Watervliet Arsenal if you want to check out the country's oldest—and still operating—weapons plant. On Dyke Avenue in Cohoes you cross marshland associated with the Mohawk River, which the trail roughly parallels from here to the end.

At about 9.5 miles, a short climb on residential Alexander Street takes you back to the railroad corridor. Here you get a bird's-eye view of the town of Colonie. The trail maintains a near-level grade in this pleasantly wooded interlude with undulating lowlands and small hillsides around you.

About a mile after Colonie Town Park, the trail briefly deviates onto quiet residential roads to navigate around Interstate 87. A short uphill takes you back to railroad grade and the trail. The first real view of the pristine Mohawk River and its wetlands at Delphus Kill comes as an awe-inspiring panorama just ahead. When you are ready to focus on the trail again, you will see woods, meadows and marshes, with occasional river vistas. The best of these is at Railroad Station Park (also called Niskayuna Lions Park) at mile 19.1. The community park is a popular trailhead, with bathrooms, picnic tables and benches. It's also a good spot to spy egrets and herons.

At mile 22.6, the trail forks, unsigned, diverging from its original alignment. Bearing left takes you on a short climb past Blatnick Park and ball field, an atomic research facility (the reason the trail diverged), and General Electric's Global Research facility before reentering the woods. Take care on this steep downhill.

By mile 26 the trail is approaching Schenectady, with urban backyards and church steeples piercing the horizon. When the trail crosses Nott Street at mile 28.4 there is a steep downgrade to the street. Once across Nott, you angle back to the rail corridor for a few blocks. The on-street portion begins at Jay Street in Little Italy. At mile 29 you enter the tree-lined Stockade Historic District with restored Victorian period homes and churches along Union Street. Go left on Church Street (be alert because trees may obscure the trail sign), to State Street and turn right. At State and Washington streets, a bus stop on the Route

55 line offers the option to return to Albany; all Capital District buses have bike racks.

Stay on State Street for two more blocks until the bike lane turns right and continues for a quarter mile while passing under Route 5. Along the way are picnic tables and a platform for viewing herons wading in the inlet and boaters on the river. Just after you pass under Route 5, the dedicated rail-trail resumes to the right. The trail here is often wooded, with glimpses of the magnificent river. Ahead is an old lock for the original Erie Canal, and at mile 32.5, Lock 8, where modern-day boaters lock through to avoid the dam. Watching them is a popular pastime, made easy with trailhead parking.

In fewer than 2 miles you're at the Rotterdam Kiwanis Park trailhead with parking, picnic tables, pit toilets, a boat launch and great river views. This park may be the best place to call it quits, as the last several miles have another on-road detour.

If you want to see the Mohawk-Hudson through, continue about a mile from the park. Leaving the trail at Mabie Lane, turn left on Pattersonville Rotterdam Junction Road (Route 5S). After about a mile turn left on Iroquois Street to return to the last short section of wooded trail.

DIRECTIONS

To reach the trailhead at Corning Riverfront Preserve, take Interstate 787 South and exit for Colonie Street. Parking and the trailhead are about a thousand feet ahead on your left.

Rotterdam Kiwanis Park provides the closest trailhead parking for the trail's west end. To reach it, from Interstate 890 take Exit 1 and travel west on Route 5S. The park and trailhead are on the right in about a thousand feet.

Contact: Capital District Transportation Committee
One Park Place
Albany, NY 12205
(518) 458-2161
www.cdtcmpo.org

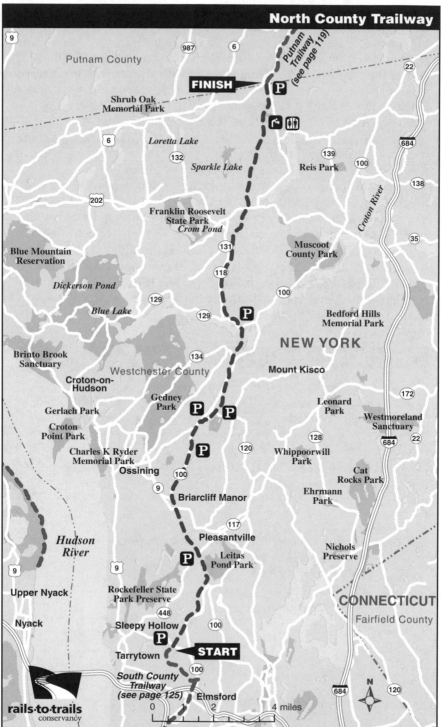

North County Trailway

Putnam County

9

987   6

Putnam Trailway (see page 119)

22

FINISH   P

Shrub Oak Memorial Park

684

6   Loretta Lake

132   Sparkle Lake

Reis Park   139   100

138

202

Franklin Roosevelt State Park   Crom Pond

Muscoot County Park

Croton River   35

Blue Mountain Reservation

131

118

Dickerson Pond

129

100

Bedford Hills Memorial Park

Blue Lake   129

129   P

NEW YORK

Brinto Brook Sanctuary

134

Westchester County

Mount Kisco

172

Croton-on-Hudson

Gedney Park   P   P

Leonard Park

Westmoreland Sanctuary

Gerlach Park

128

684   22

Croton Point Park

P

120

Whippoorwill Park

Charles K Ryder Memorial Park   Ossining   100

Cat Rocks Park

9

Briarcliff Manor

Ehrmann Park

117

Hudson River

Pleasantville

Nichols Preserve

9   P   9   Leitas Pond Park

Upper Nyack

Rockefeller State Park Preserve

CONNECTICUT
Fairfield County

Nyack

448

Sleepy Hollow   100   P

Tarrytown   **START**

South County Trailway (see page 125)   100

684   120

rails·to·trails
conservancy

Elmsford

0   2   4 miles

N

North County Trailway

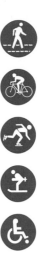

The North County Trailway is the longest of the four connected rail-trails breathing new life into the former New York Central Railroad's Putnam Division line. The "Old Put" provided passenger and freight service between New York City and Brewster, in Putnam County, from the 1880s. Passenger service ended in 1958 and freight services ended in 1980.

The trail spans 22.1 miles in Westchester County. From Mount Pleasant (where it becomes the South County Trailway, see page 125, on its southward trek to the New York City line) the trailway extends north to the Putnam County border where it seamlessly transitions into the Putnam Trailway (see page 119) rolling 9.7 miles north. From Old Saw Mill River Road at the North County Trailway's southern end, the trail runs parallel to the high-traffic Saw Mill River Parkway on the right and woodlands and a power transmission corridor on the left. After crossing over Old Saw Mill River Road,

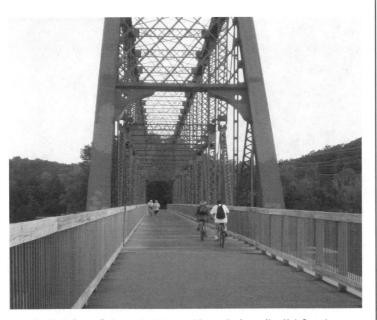

The North County Trailway is breathing new life into the former New York Central Railroad's Putnam Division line.

Location
Westchester County

Endpoints
Old Saw Mill River Road in Mount Pleasant to Baldwin Place Road in Somers

Mileage
22.1

Roughness Index
1

Surface
Asphalt

there is a side trail on the left that leads down to a parking lot along the road. The trail then crosses State Route 117, Bedford Road, on a bridge. Highway traffic is never far away from this southern section of the trail, but a narrow strip of trees provides welcome shade and screening from the traffic.

Just beyond Pleasantville Road is a side trail to the Tudor-style Briarcliff Library, formerly the Briarcliff Manor train station. Then you hit the first of two on-road detours: Saw Mill River Road, which parallels the trail corridor here, provides a wide shoulder for the short distance to Chappaqua Road when the rail-trail returns and runs you through the woods between Saw Mill River Road and the Taconic State Parkway.

Your second journey on the shoulder of Saw Mill River Road begins at the intersection of North State Road. This 0.75-mile detour takes you past Echo Lake State Park and over the Taconic State Parkway before the North County Trailway resumes on rail corridor. The trail through Millwood looks out on commercial and industrial buildings before crossing Millwood Road and entering a wooded stretch.

About 0.75 mile of this wooded area is the edge of Kitchawan Preserve. This sprawling property on New Croton Reservoir that was once a research facility of the Brooklyn Botanic Garden now has miles of hiking trails to explore. Staying straight on the rail-trail brings you

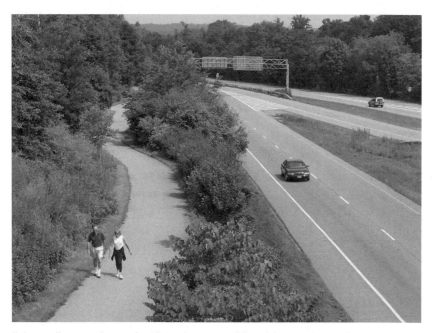

Highway traffic is never far away from the southern section of the trail, but a narrow strip of trees provides welcome shade and screening from the traffic.

to a bridge over an arm of the reservoir that supplies water to New York City.

In the village of Yorktown Heights shops, including boutiques, galleries and jewelers, as well as restaurants, ranging from fast food to delis to cafes, are only a block off the trail. Shortly after leaving the village the trail crosses Saw Mill River Road—this time at a steep grade, so be cautious. Beyond Granite Springs Road a large orchard signals the trail's transition to a more agricultural and forested setting for its final 6 miles. The trail ends in Somers at Baldwin Place when you emerge from the woods.

The Putman Trailway begins when you cross Route 118 (Tomahawk Street). Parking here is adjacent to a shopping center that contains a number of restaurants.

DIRECTIONS

Parking for the southern end of the trail in Mount Pleasant is in the Eastview Park and Ride Lot. Take Saw Mill River Parkway to Exit 23 for Eastview. Follow Old Saw Mill River Road west until it becomes Neperan Road. The park and ride lot is on the right side of the road.

To reach the Somers trailhead, from the Taconic State Parkway take US Route 6 east. Bear right onto State Route 118. Turn right onto the Somers Commons Shopping Center access road. A dirt parking lot for the trail is on the left. A dirt path leads up to the trail.

Contact: Westchester County Department of Parks and Recreation
25 Monroe Street
Mt. Kisco, NY 10549
(914) 864-PARK (7275)
www.westchestergov.com/parks

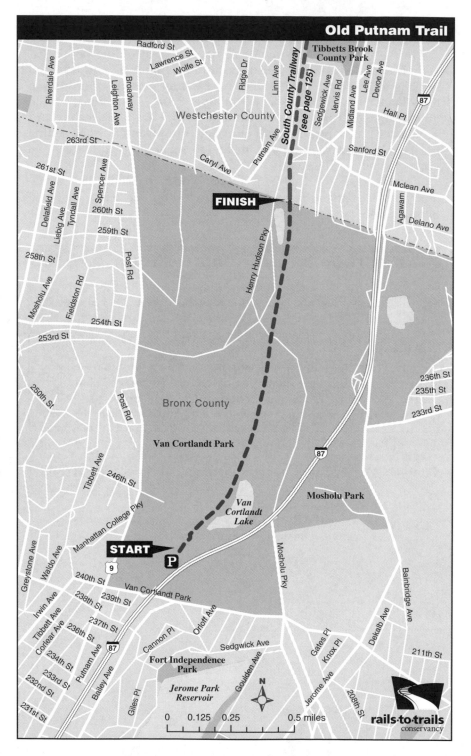

Old Putnam Trail

Old Putnam Trail

Splayed over 1,146 acres in northwest Bronx, Van Cortlandt Park has a lot going on. The park is New York City's fourth largest and is home to the oldest municipal golf course in the U.S. There are playgrounds, walking trails, running tracks, scores of ball fields, a nature center, a museum and scenic freshwater lake. Van Cortlandt Park also is home to the Old Putnam Trail, one of four rail-trails on the former New York Central Railroad's Putnam Division line. The wide dirt and grass corridor allows easy passage on foot or by bicycle.

Access the trail from the northwest corner of the large parking lot near the Van Cortlandt Golf House. Though a portion of rail corridor extends south from here, it is heavily overgrown. Head south from the entrance a short distance to see the remnants of an old passenger platform. All that remains is the rusted metal framework.

The trail's best scenery and its most unusual sight are immediate. The trail skirts Van Cortlandt Lake and then passes 13 large stones along the west side of the corridor. Railroad baron Commodore Cornelius Vanderbilt had these stone slabs shipped from quarries to determine which would be best (most impervious to weathering) for building Grand Central Station in New

Location
Bronx County

Endpoints
Van Cortlandt Park to Westchester County Line in New York City

Mileage
1.25

Roughness Index
2

Surface
Cinder, dirt and grass

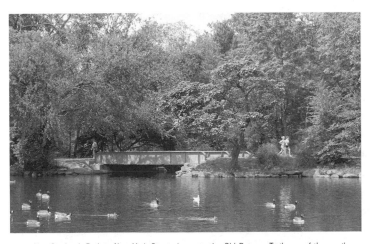

Van Cortlandt Park in New York City is home to the Old Putnam Trail, one of three rail-trails on the former New York Central Railroad's Putnam Division line.

York City. Despite the results of his experiment, Indiana limestone was chosen because it was cheaper to transport. The Indiana limestone sample is the second southernmost stone in this lineup.

As you continue north you pass several trails that connect to the John Kiernan Nature Trail. This 1.25-mile trail named for a Bronx naturalist meanders by Van Cortlandt Lake, a wetland and the forest. Staying on the Old Putnam Trail brings you over a small bridge spanning an arm of Van Cortlandt Lake. Across the lake are views of the Bronx skyline and the golf course clubhouse.

At the Westchester County line, the Old Putnam Trail gives way to the South County Trailway (see page 125). This asphalt paved trail extends 2.35 miles to Redmond Park in Yonkers. Here there is a 2.1-mile break in the South County Trailway that can be navigated on surface streets.

DIRECTIONS

To reach Van Cortlandt Park in the Bronx, from Broadway/US Route 9 go east onto Van Cortlandt Park South. Turn left at the second light and bear to the left, following signs for Van Cortlandt Golf Course, to a large parking lot. At the far end of the parking lot on the left side is a pathway that leads to the Old Putnam Trail.

To reach the Old Putman Trail via the South County Trailway in Yonkers, from Central Park Avenue in Yonkers, exit at Palmer Road and travel west to Mile Square Road (traffic light) and turn left. Proceed south on Mile Square Road to Cook Avenue. Turn right and drive south on Cook Avenue to the entrance to Redmond Park on the right. Turn right into the park and proceed to the parking lot. A paved ramp leads up to the trail at the far end of the parking lot.

Contact: City of New York Department of Parks and Recreation
The Arsenal, Central Park
830 Fifth Avenue
New York, NY 10065
311 in NYC, (212) NEW-YORK
  or (212) 639-9675 outside NYC
www.nycgovparks.org/parks/VanCortlandtPark

Friends of Van Cortlandt Park
124 Gale Place, Apt. GrndA
Bronx, NY 10463
(718) 601-1553
www.vancortlandt.org

Ontario Pathways Rail Trail

Shaped like a left-leaning V, the Ontario Pathways Rail Trail travels southwest from Canandaigua to Stanley, then shoots north to Clifton Springs. The rural trail is the pride of an industrious community organization, Ontario Pathways, Inc., that purchased the unused railroad corridor and transformed it into a popular recreation destination. Nineteen miles of the rail-trail are open, and ten of twelve bridges have been redecked or rebuilt. One of the bridges at the Canandaigua end is enhanced with a decorative metal gate in the shape of the organization's logo and name. A similar gate is in place in Clifton Springs.

For the first few miles in Canandaigua, an active rail line is separated from the trail by a thick, overgrown hedgerow. The trail's surface is single track, occasionally wider, of packed cinder ballast bordered by mowed grass and trees.

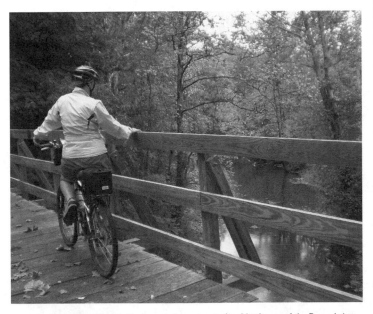

An enormously pleasant ride through the vast agricultural landscape of the Finger Lakes Region, the Ontario Pathways Rail Trail features 10 rebuilt bridges.

Location
Ontario County

Endpoints
Canandaigua to
Clifton Springs

Mileage
19

Roughness Index
3

Surface
Cinder and grass

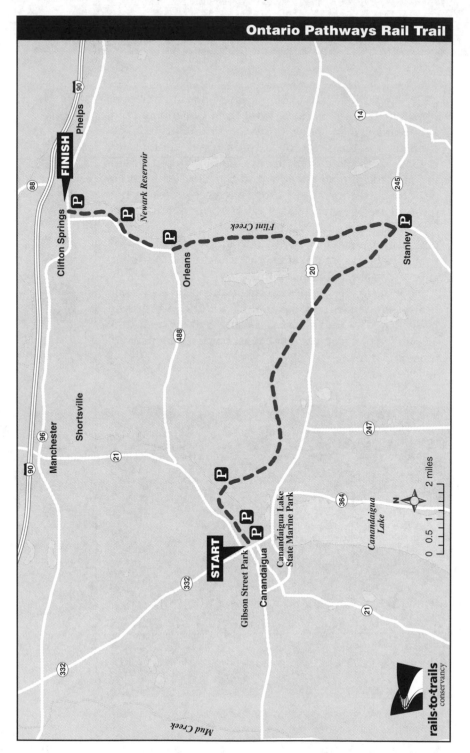

Ontario Pathways Rail Trail

It's an enormously pleasant ride through the vast agricultural landscape of the Finger Lakes Region passing acres and acres of green cabbage, red cabbage, squash, celery, soybeans and corn. If you ride the trail often enough, you will witness the full cycle of America's produce being grown and harvested.

At the Orleans Trailhead, along County Road 23, is a railroad water tower. The wooden tank, which held 40,000 gallons, is one of a few of the remaining towers that serviced steam locomotives throughout the Northeast.

At this point there is a break in the trail that requires on-road navigation to reach the last section of rail-trail north of Clifton Springs. It is worth the extra effort to enjoy the northernmost segment's beautiful waterfalls and nicely constructed bridges.

Be sure to budget enough time to explore the quaint town of Canandaigua perched on the north shore of Canandaigua Lake, one of the smaller of New York's Finger Lakes. With loads of Victorian architecture and a population of fewer than 15,000, Canandaigua has the essence of a tiny resort town. From June through October you can tour historic neighborhoods and a hilltop cemetery in horse-drawn carriages. A replica 19th-century paddleboat offers dinner cruises. In town, local entertainment and art provide a counterpoint to gorgeous views across the lake and valley, dotted with produce farms and vineyards.

DIRECTIONS

From Interstate 90, exit onto Route 332 South into the town of Canandaigua. Turn left onto Ontario Street and travel one block to the municipal parking lot on the left.

To reach the Orleans Trailhead, from Interstate 90, take Exit 43 to head south on Route 21/N. Main Street. Turn left to head east on Route 488. Turn right on Waddell Road/Railroad Avenue. A small parking lot is on the left, just prior to reaching County Road 23.

Contact: Ontario Pathways
P.O. Box 996
Canandaigua, NY 14424
(585) 234-7722
www.ontariopathways.org

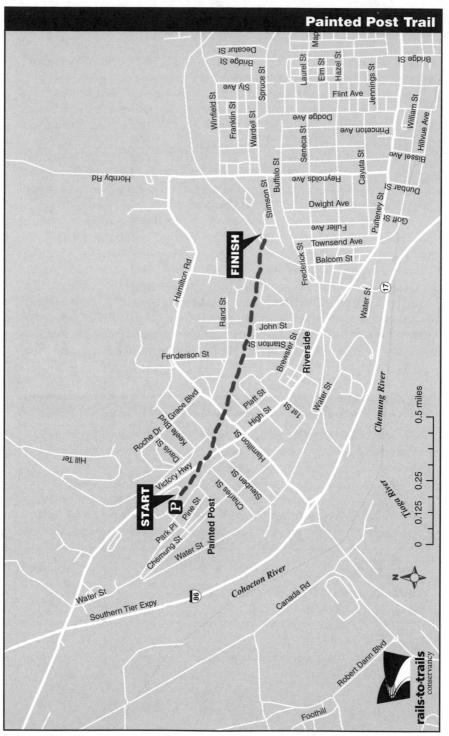

Painted Post Trail

Painted Post Trail

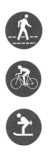

If you are near Corning, New York, and need a nice walk, check out this charming respite. The Painted Post Trail connects schools, playgrounds, other trails, and residential neighborhoods west of Corning. The wide right-of-way (nearly 100 feet) accommodates the trail's interesting design: Instead of following the straight line of the railroad track, the trail gently weaves through a grassy park setting.

The trail begins just past the community swimming pool in Craig Park, named for former village Mayor Charles Craig. The park has basketball and tennis courts, a sand volleyball court, a skateboard park, and numerous picnic tables and grills. The rail-trail passes some homes before shooting through an underpass of the combination Victoria Highway and New York Route 415.

A restored railroad depot sits along the trail near Steuben Street. It serves as a railroad museum staffed

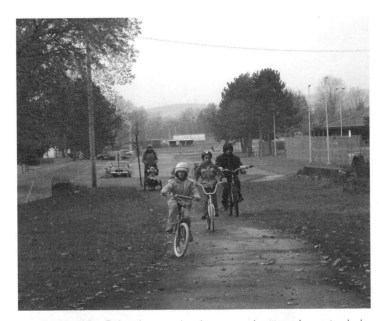

The Painted Post Trail gently weaves through a grassy park setting and connects schools, playgrounds, other trails and residential neighborhoods.

Location
Yates County

Endpoints
Painted Post to Riverside

Mileage
1.1

Roughness Index
2

Surface
Cinder

113

by volunteers. After crossing Steuben Street the trail skirts the High Street Cemetery. A bridge takes you over a small creek then the trail goes under Interstate 86 and ends at the intersection of Western Lane and Cutler Avenue.

The Painted Post Trail is a vital part of the community. Many events are held along the trail throughout the year including the well-known Wineglass Marathon, which has been taking place for several decades.

DIRECTIONS

To reach the trailhead in Craig Park, from Interstate 86 take Route 15 to Exit 43 on the west side of Corning. Exit east onto High Street (toward Corning and Painted Post). Pass West High School and turn right immediately onto a drive that leads into Craig Park. Follow the road past the swimming pool, through the parking area and to the trailhead.

Contact: Painted Post Parks & Recreation
P. O. Box 110
Village of Painted Post, NY 14870
(607) 962-4605
www.paintedpostny.com/index.html

Pat McGee Trail

M ake way for diversity on the Pat McGee Trail. This 12.1-mile path boasts a diverse array of plant and animal life, with more than 150 species of birds. A variety of users, including snowmobilers and equestrians, can be seen. The trail even crosses the Eastern Continental Divide, meaning that the rainfall on one end of the trail is diverted to the Atlantic Ocean and on the other end to the Gulf of Mexico.

The trail connects seven quiet communities in the heart of Cattaraugus County in southwest New York. If you begin your journey at the northern trailhead just south of Cattaraugus, be prepared for a climb. The grade is gentle but you will know you are going uphill. Not far from the trailhead is a lean-to. Snowmobile riders huddle here in winter months, and in summer it provides relief from sudden storms. The rail-trail's first several miles pass mostly through woodland as you climb toward the Eastern Continental Divide. Informational signs chronicle the wide assortment of mammals (41 species) and plants (174 species), as well as describe geological features and 9 unique ecosystems. In spring the woods abound with wildflowers. Keep an eye out for white-tailed deer and other wildlife on the trail ahead.

After passing the Eastern Continental Divide, the trail begins a slight descent and the landscape changes

Location
Cattaraugus County

Endpoints
Cattaraugus to Salamanca

Mileage
12.1

Roughness Index
2

Surface
Crushed stone

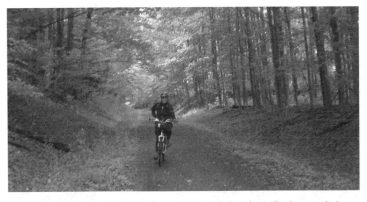

The Pat McGee Trail's first several miles pass mostly through woodland as you climb toward the Eastern Continental Divide.

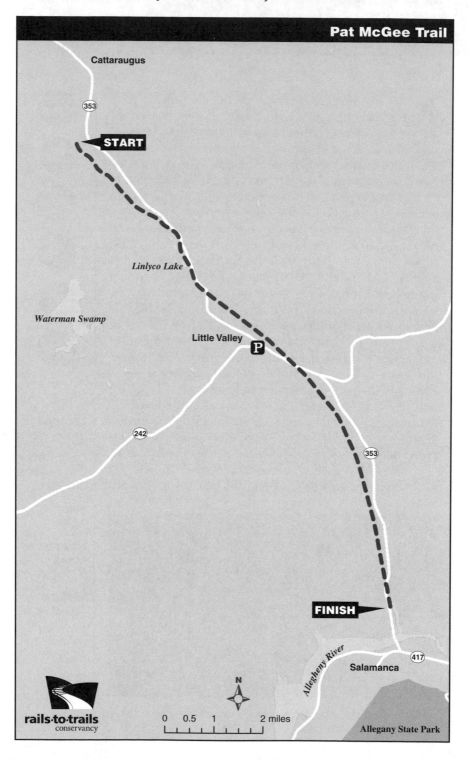

Pat McGee Trail

Cattaraugus

353

START

Linlyco Lake

Waterman Swamp

Little Valley P

242

353

FINISH

Allegheny River

Salamanca

417

Allegany State Park

N

rails·to·trails
conservancy

0   0.5   1   2 miles

to wetlands. There is agricultural activity here, too, signaling the rural nature of the communities woven together by this old rail line.

In the village of Little Valley, about midway on your journey, a community recreational park has pavilions and picnic tables. Didn't pack your picnic lunch? Head a block or two into the village where shops and eateries welcome trail visitors. A short paved section of trail leads from the park southward.

Other trails cross and branch off of the Pat McGee Trail. These trails are used by snowmobilers, hikers and equestrians. The North Country National Scenic Trail, Bi-Centennial Bike Trail and the Finger Lakes Trail provide additional opportunities to enjoy scenic Cattaraugus County.

The southern section of the Pat McGee Trail travels through farmland with wide vistas of the surrounding hills. Six railroad bridges over several streams have been restored for trail use. There are big plans and a multi-phase strategy to connect the rail-trail with Allegany State Park, Zoar Valley natural area, Erie County to the north, and two of the Seneca Nation of Indians' reservations. For now, the only connections are with the DEC Trail, primarily an equestrian trail and the Finger Lakes Hiking Trail. Both trails connect to the rail-trail south of Little Valley.

The trail is named for Patricia McGee, the longtime state senator from nearby Franklinville who championed the trail project. When the senator passed away in 2005, there was unanimous support for naming the new trail in her honor.

DIRECTIONS

To reach the northern endpoint, just south of Cattaraugus on State Route 353, turn onto Leon Road (County Road #6). The trail begins on the left side of the road. There is limited parking on the right side of the road.

To reach the southern endpoint, from Interstate 86, take the exit for New York State Route 417. Proceed east on Route 417. Turn left onto New York State Route 353, or Center Street. Just north of Salamanca, on the right side of Route 353, you will see parking and the start of the Pat McGee Trail.

Contact: Cattaraugus Local Development Corporation
P.O. Box 1
Cattaraugus, NY 14719
(716) 257-3237
www.cldc.net

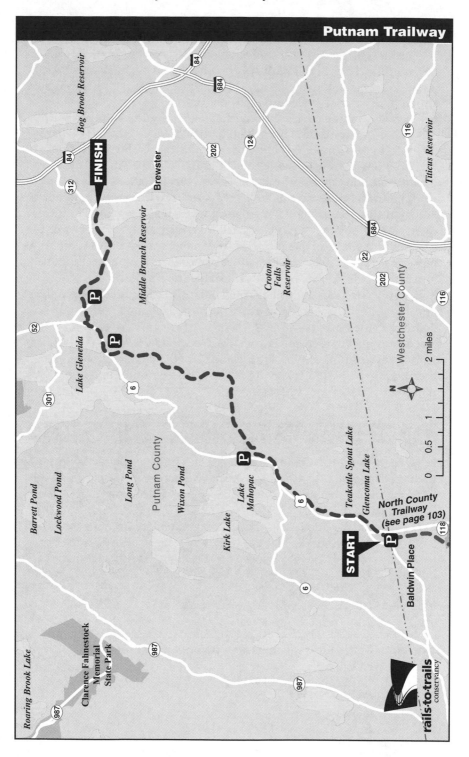

Putnam Trailway

Putnam Trailway

The final passenger cars of the Putnam Division of the New York Central Railroad ran in 1958, but the rail line that so influenced development of this area still sparks nostalgia. The "Old Put" carried commuters from New York City north to Brewster where connections took travelers to Boston and Montreal. Freight service for farm products from rural areas of Putnam and Westchester counties continued until the 1980s.

Nearly 45 miles of the "Old Put" corridor, from Van Cortlandt Park in New York City north to Putnam County, have been converted into four connecting rail-trails. The Putnam Trailway is the northernmost of the trails atop the train line. Currently 10.9 miles are open for public use from the Putnam County line at Baldwin Place, where Westchester County's North County Trailway (see page 103) terminates, to Putnam Avenue in Brewster.

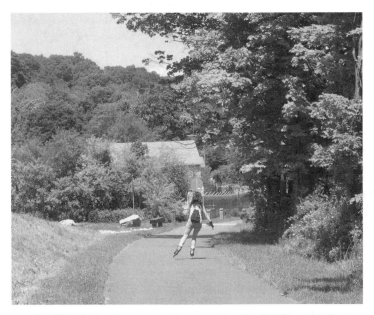

The "Old Put" railroad line once carried commuters from New York City north to Brewster, but 45 miles have been converted into four connecting rail-trails.

Location
Putnam County

Endpoints
Route 118 in Somers (between Route 6 and the intersection of Miller Road and Tomahawk Street) to Old Mine Road in Tilly Foster

Mileage
10.9

Roughness Index
1

Surface
Asphalt

North from Baldwin Place is a gentle uphill slope. Busy Route 6 is just to the west, and a residential development flanks the east side of the trail. As you briefly enter a wooded area, Bloomer Pond appears on your right. Bucks Hollow Road runs adjacent to the trail here, providing several access points. The hamlet of Mahopac provides additional opportunities to access the trail. Past Croton Falls Road the trail edges and enters a mixed hardwood forest for the 1.7 miles to Lake Casse. The woods are busy with squirrels and chipmunks constantly looking for food and shelter. Many bird species live in these woods. Their calls can be heard throughout the day.

To take in the view at Lake Casse, hop off the trail at Lake Road. After Lake Casse, the rail-trail descends and plunges into a dense forest. On the outskirts of the hamlet of Carmel, the trail runs along Route 6 again with the south bank of Lake Gleneida on the far side of the road. Swimming in this water supply lake is prohibited, but in winter warmly dressed anglers cluster around their ice fishing holes. Warm weather fishing and boating are also permitted here.

A 1.2-mile extension added in 2010 carries the trail farther north to Putnam Avenue. The final 0.9-mile section to North Main Street in Brewster will be completed by 2012.

DIRECTIONS

To reach the Somers Trailhead, from the Taconic Parkway, exit for US Route 6 East. At Baldwin Place turn right onto State Route 118. Parking for the trail is off of the second entrance into Somers Commons Shopping Center.

To reach the Old Mine Road Trailhead in Tilly Foster, from Interstate 84, take Exit 19 to State Route 312. Proceed west on Route 312 for approximately 1 mile. At the intersection of Route 312 and US Route 6 (Carmel Avenue), proceed straight. Turn left onto Tilly Foster Road. Trailhead parking is on the right.

Contact: Putnam County Planning Department
841 Fair Street
Carmel, NY 10512
(845) 878-3480
www.putnamcountyny.com/planning/index.htm

Rochester, Syracuse and Eastern Trail

The town of Perinton, New York, has been hard at work improving the Rochester, Syracuse and Eastern Trail, and it shows. Since 1996, when the American Hiking Society designated Perinton as a Trail Town USA, the trail has a new connection with the town hall and its surrounding park facilities, and there is a state-of-the-art road crossing at busy Route 31. Even the crushed limestone surface is in great shape.

The rail-trail connects with the town's Crescent Trail footpath system and is in sight of the Erie Canal trail between Buffalo and Albany. Known alternately as the RS&E Trail, the Perinton Hike/Bikeway Trail, or the Trolley Trail (for the electric trolley that ran on the corridor), it provides an excellent spot for a walk or bike ride.

Start your adventure at Egypt Park on the corner of Route 31 and Victor Road. From the southwest corner of the parking lot, follow a short connecting path to the trail. Turn right onto the rail-trail, but look left to see the horses and other animals of Lollypop Farms, the large

Location
Monroe County

Endpoints
Egypt Park in Perinton and NY State Barge Canal

Mileage
3

Roughness Index
1

Surface
Crushed stone

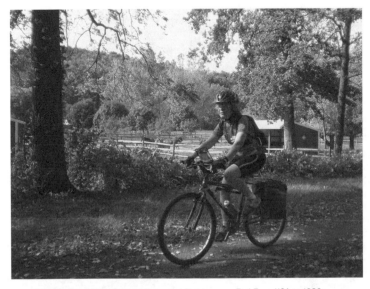

The American Hiking Society designated Perinton as a Trail Town USA in 1996.

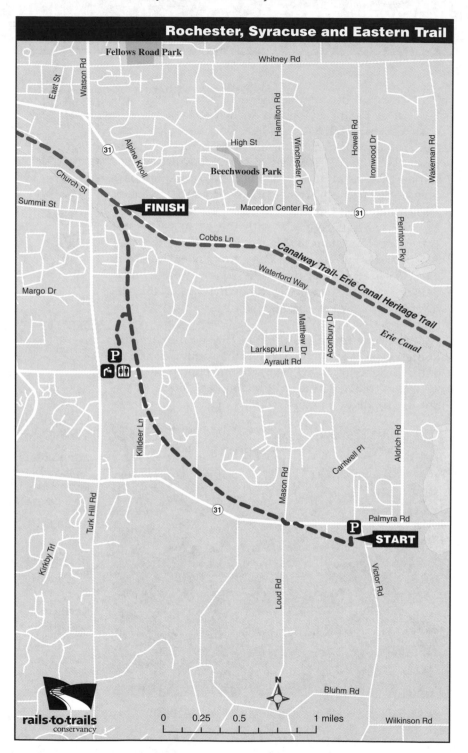

Human Society branch of Monroe and Rochester counties. If you have time at the end of the trip, visit their education center, hands-on outdoor pens or even the adoption center.

At the half-mile mark the trail crosses Route 31. At the far side of the busy road, the trail continues on the left. You may notice the power lines overhead. The Rochester, Syracuse and Eastern Trail is one of the many rail-trails—nearly 40 percent—that pulls double duty as a recreation and transportation corridor and a utility right-of-way.

You may feel the headwind off Lake Ontario, about 10 miles north, after crossing over Route 31. If you listen closely, you can hear the train whistle from the active rail line a few miles still ahead. Forested and open wetlands buffer the trail for much of its length, and at times the trail rises 15 feet. The trail winds its way through neighborhoods and connects with some backyards. You will see parents pushing baby strollers in the late morning and kids walking home from school in the later afternoon.

At 2.3 miles a new connecting trail will take you 0.25 mile up the hill to the Perinton Town Hall and Community Center complex and park. At the base of the hill on the connecting trail are nice soccer fields, a storm shelter, bathrooms and picnic areas. Farther up, at the top of the hill, you will see a pool and indoor waterslide.

Once back on the rail-trail turn left. The trail continues for another two-thirds of a mile and then ends abruptly at a guardrail overlooking the Erie Canal. Unfortunately it doesn't connect to the canal's towpath, but folks back at the Perinton Town Hall are happy to provide on-road directions to the towpath so you can keep enjoying this Trail Town USA.

DIRECTIONS

To reach the Egypt Park Trailhead, from Interstate 490 take Exit 26 to Route 31 east. Continue on Route 31 and Pittsford-Palmyra Road for almost 4 miles until you see Egypt Park on your right. At the intersection of Mason and Loud roads, the trail crosses Route 31, but travel another half mile and turn right on Victor Road. Turn right again into the Egypt Park parking area.

Contact: Recreation and Parks Department
1350 Turk Hill Road
Fairport, NY 14450
(585) 223-5050
www.perinton.org/Departments/RandP

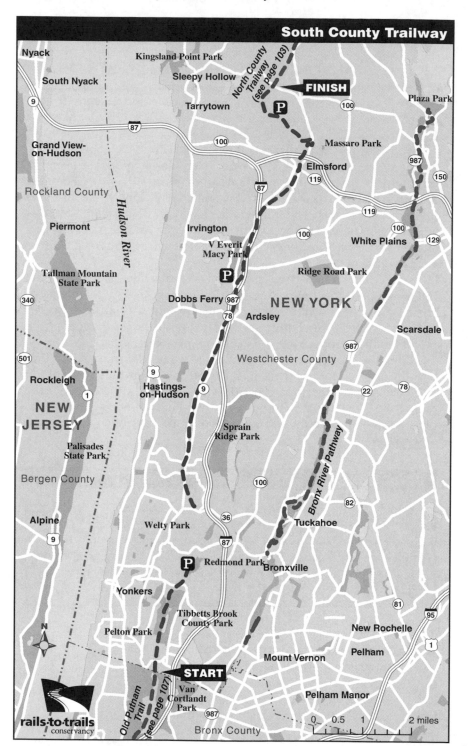

South County Trailway

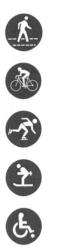

The South County Trailway is a zippy paved trail heading north from Yonkers through the Hudson River Valley communities of Hastings-on-Hudson, Dobbs Ferry, Ardsley, Irvington, Greenburgh and Elmsford. Popular with bike commuters seeking relief from the area's busy streets and parkways, the trail follows the former Putnam Division line of the New York Central Railroad, and links two other rail-trails on the same line: the Old Putnam Trail (see page 107) in the south and the North County Trailway (see page 103) in Mount Pleasant. Two unfinished sections require on-road detours, though one, in Elmsford, will be resolved shortly.

The trail begins at the border of Westchester County and New York City, just outside Van Cortlandt Park. However, there is no trail access at this location. You must approach either from the Old Putnam Trail out of Van Cortlandt Park or by proceeding south from Redmond Park.

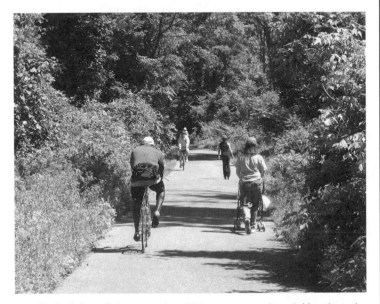

The South County Trailway is popular with bike commuters seeking relief from the area's busy streets and parkways.

Location
Westchester County

Endpoints
Redmond Park in Yonkers to Old Saw Mill River Road in Mount Pleasant

Mileage
14.1

Roughness Index
1

Surface
Asphalt

North from Redmond Park, there is a 2.1-mile break in the trail. Following roads and signed bike lanes or shoulders will bring you to Tuckahoe Road where the trail resumes. Leave Redmond Park and turn right onto Cook Avenue. Take a slight left onto Mile Square Road. Mile Square Road intersects with Tuckahoe Road. Turn left onto Tuckahoe Road. Turn right onto Touissant Avenue and pick up the trail on the left.

The next 7.5 miles are smooth sailing; the trail passes through mixed residential and commercial areas and parallels the Saw Mill River Parkway. Through V. Everit Macy Park the trail runs between the parkway and the New York Thruway. Though the majority is bordered by a fencerow of deciduous trees and brush, you are seldom far from traffic noise. The numerous side road crossings are well signed, but be alert at all crossings both for motorists and cyclists.

In Elmsford, another short gap in the rail-trail requires on-road navigation. The Route 9A Bypass Project will eventually eliminate this half-mile detour. When the trail ends at Main Street in Elmsford, turn right to cross Main Street at the traffic light. Turn left and then turn right through the parking lot to Vreeland Avenue. Follow Vreeland Avenue through a commercial and industrial area and make a slight right onto Hayes Street. Hayes Street turns right and becomes North Payne Street. At the stop sign, turn left onto Saw Mill River Road.

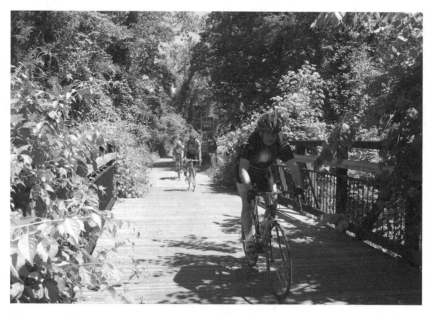

A fencerow of deciduous trees and brush borders much of the trail.

Turn left onto Warehouse Lane, which dead-ends where the South County Trailway resumes.

The official endpoint of the South County Trailway, and the start of the 22-mile North County Trailway, is where the corridor crosses Old Saw Mill River Road. If you want to extend—or even double— your mileage, cross the road and make tracks on the line where the Old Put ran.

DIRECTIONS

To reach Redmond Park in Yonkers, from Central Park Avenue in Yonkers, exit at Palmer Road and travel west to Mile Square Road (traffic light) and turn left. Proceed south on Mile Square Road to Cook Avenue. Turn right and drive south on Cook Avenue to the entrance to Redmond Park on the right. Turn right into the park and proceed to the parking lot. A paved ramp leads up to the trail at the far end of the parking lot.

To reach Touissant Avenue in Yonkers, from Interstate 87 take the Tuckahoe Road exit to go east on Tuckahoe Road. Turn right onto Touissant Avenue. The trail is on the right. There is limited street parking on this short residential road.

To reach Mount Pleasant, take Saw Mill River Parkway to Exit 23 for Eastview. Follow Old Saw Mill River Road west until it becomes Neperan Road. The park and ride lot is on the right side of the road. Parking for the northern end of the trail is in the Eastview Park and Ride Lot.

Contact: Westchester County Department of Parks and Recreation
25 Monroe Street
Mt. Kisco, NY 10549
(914) 864-PARK (7275)
www.westchestergov.com/parks

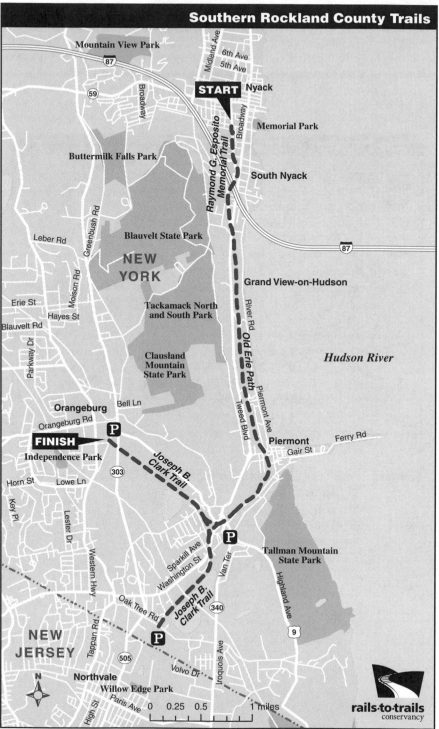

Southern Rockland County Trails

These three contiguous trails—the Raymond G. Esposito Memorial Trail, Old Erie Path and Joseph B. Clark Trail—occupy the former right-of-way of the Erie Railroad's Nyack and Piermont Branch. Each trail is fairly short but taken together they make for a wonderful experience along the banks of the Hudson River.

The Raymond G. Esposito Memorial Trail in South Nyack, named for a late mayor of this village, is a milelong gravel trail through several neighborhoods on the Hudson River. From its start in a community park, the rail-trail heads south, occasionally high above some of the neighborhoods it passes. Extensive stairways on the steep slopes have been constructed to connect residents with the rail-trail. The trail runs parallel to South Franklin Street crossing Brookside and Clinton avenues. These are low-volume residential roads, but trail users should stop at each intersection before proceeding. The

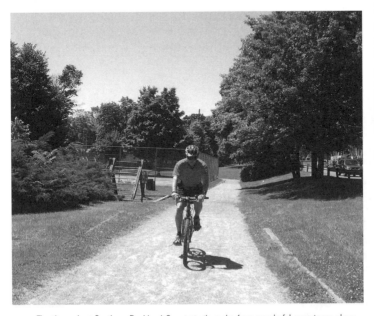

The three short Southern Rockland County trails make for a wonderful experience along the banks of the Hudson River.

Location
Rockland County

Endpoints
South Franklin Street and Cedar Hill Avenue in South Nyack to Oak Tree Road in Tappan to Greenbush Road in Orangeburg

Mileage
6.8

Roughness Index
2

Surface
Asphalt, dirt, grass and gravel

129

trail crosses over the New York State Thruway on the original railroad bridge, redecked for trail use. By the time you touch down on the far side of the highway, at South Broadway Avenue, the Esposito Trail ends and the Old Erie Path begins.

The 3-mile Old Erie Path has a rougher surface than the Esposito Trail, but is suitable for walking and for hybrid or mountain biking. In contrast to the prior mile along roads and homes, this path is more remote. The railroad bed was cut into the side of steep hillsides that drop into the Hudson River, so trail users have a spectacular view across the wide river. Home owners, many of them high above or downhill from the corridor, access the trail by way of creative engineering: You will see hillside stairways with handrails fashioned from the limbs of native trees, as well as decorative archways and gates on intricate pulley systems.

In Piermont the trail curves west away from the river. Just before the trail crosses Hudson Terrace, you'll find the restored Piermont train station, which houses information on the area's railroad history. Then the Old Erie Path begins a milelong, densely wooded, gentle descent into the town of Sparkill, where it meets the 2.8-mile Joseph B. Clark Trail.

In Sparkill Park you must choose between following the Clark Trail 1.5 miles north and west (turn right) or 1.3 miles south (turn left). Heading south the rail-trail passes behind a residential neighborhood before entering a forested area. The trail crosses Sparkill Avenue and Washington Street. Both trail users and motorists are made aware of the crossings by the use of red pavers. After passing under the Palisades Interstate Parkway the trail continues through woodlands ending at Oak Tree Road.

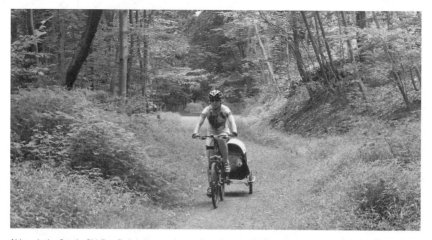

Although the 3-mile Old Erie Path has a rougher surface than the Esposito Trail, it is suitable for walking and for hybrid or mountain biking.

Backtracking to Sparkill Park the remainder of the Joseph B. Clark Trail heads toward Orangeburg. After crossing Kings Highway, the trail leaves the village and enters a forested landscape. A bridge carries the trail over Sparkill Creek. A pedestrian bridge carries the trail over busy New York Route 303. The paved trail ends at Greenbush Road in Orangeburg.

DIRECTIONS

To reach the South Nyack endpoint, from the New York State Thruway (Interstates 87 and 287), take Exit 11. Southbound traffic will be on New York Route 59, Main Street. (Thruway traffic northbound will exit onto High Avenue. Turn right on North Highland Avenue, and then turn left onto Main Street.) From Main Street in South Nyack turn right on South Franklin Street. The trail begins in the park at the corner of South Franklin Street and Cedar Hill Avenue. There is only on-street parking available.

To reach the Oak Tree Road endpoint in Tappan, from the Palisades Interstate Parkway, take Exit 5 South to U.S. Route 303. Turn left onto Oak Tree Road. There is a small parking lot on the left for trail users.

To reach the Greenbush Road endpoint in Orangeburg, from the Palisades Interstate Parkway, take Exit 6 East onto County Route 20, West Orangeburg Road. Turn right onto County Route 15/Western Highway. Turn left onto Highview Avenue. Turn right onto Greenbush Road. Enter the Lowes store parking lot. There is parking for trail users in the northeast corner of the parking lot.

Contact: Joseph B. Clark Trail and Old Erie Path:
Orangetown Parks and Recreation Department
81 Hunt Road
Orangeburg, NY 10962
(854) 359-6503
www.orangetown.com

Raymond G. Esposito Memorial Trail:
Village of South Nyack
282 South Broadway
South Nyack, NY 10960
(845) 358-0244
www.southnyack.info

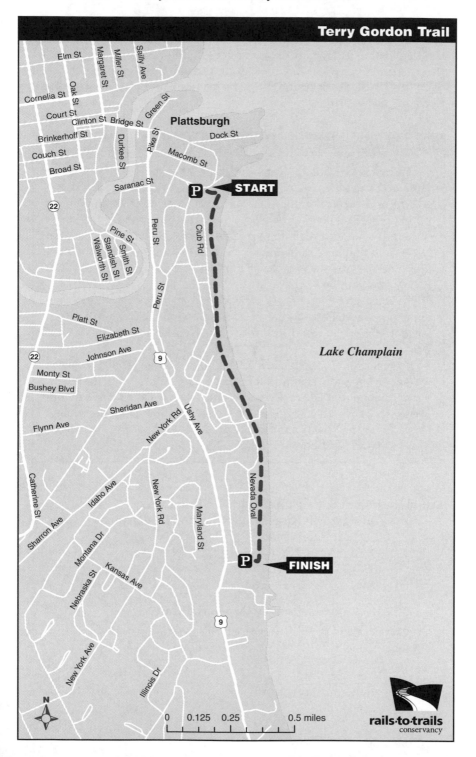

Terry Gordon Trail

Plattsburgh

Lake Champlain

START

FINISH

Terry Gordon Trail

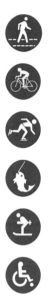

Tthis multi-use community trail is a hit with locals, and it appeals to visitors—especially those with a yen for military history. Plattsburgh, New York, has figured in this country's war history from the American Revolution and the War of 1812 to the Cold War.

The Terry Gordon Trail (also known as the Terry James Gordon Recreational Path) is part of Plattsburgh's developing network of on- and off-street bike routes and a river walk. Built adjacent to the Canadian Pacific Railway's still-active main line along Lake Champlain, this rail-with-trail begins with a magnificent view of the lake and the Green Mountains of Vermont in the distance. Near the start, a stone monument dedicates the trail to Terry James Gordon, CITY COUNCILOR, COURT CLERK, HISTORIAN, RUNNER.

Traveling south, you'll be tantalized by glimpses of sparkling Lake Champlain to your left, while on your right you have a clear view of the community. Watch for the buildings of the U.S. Oval National Historic District, formerly Plattsburgh Air Force Base, which closed in 1995. The brick dwellings that once housed high-ranking officers are now private homes. At mile 0.9 you'll see the old stone U.S. Armed Forces Barracks, built in 1820. Ulysses S. Grant lived in one of these while stationed here as an army lieutenant. Just beyond, an overpass connects to the lakefront and a fishing pier.

At trail's end you can return the way you came. Or, better yet, vary your route by following bike route signs north mostly off-road and along U.S. Route 9 to Clyde Lewis Park. You'll see an old cemetery that is well worth exploring, signs for the War of 1812 Museum, and the venerable barracks from a different vantage point. Then cross the park to pick up the rail-with-trail and return to your starting point.

To make a day of it, get your hands on a map of Plattsburgh's connecting bike routes and historic attractions. Contact the Community Development Office (listed below) for a map.

Location
Clinton County

Endpoints
Intersection of Jay and Hamilton streets to Nevada Oval East in Plattsburgh

Mileage
1.6

Roughness Index
1

Surface
Asphalt

DIRECTIONS

To reach the northern endpoint, from Interstate 87, take Exit 36 and follow State Route 22 for about 2.5 miles until you reach a fork. Take the right fork at South Peru Street and go about 0.8 mile to U.S. Route 9. Follow Route 9 north about 0.5 mile. Turn right onto Hamilton Street and follow it for two blocks. The trail begins on your right, with a few street parking spots at the trailhead.

Contact: Community Development Office
41 City Hall Place
Plattsburgh, NY 12901
(518) 563-7642
www.cityofplattsburgh.com

Uncle Sam Bike Trail

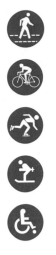

Inland and east of the Hudson River, the Uncle Sam Bike Trail (also called the Uncle Sam Trail or Uncle Sam Bikeway) largely serves as a trail for residents of Troy. If, however, you are traveling in the area and want to stretch your legs, this trail offers a scenic retreat. It is also part of the extensive network of trails and on-road bike routes in the area. All of these appear on the Mohawk-Hudson Bike-Hike Trail map (see page 99), free from the Capital District Transportation Authority.

For convenient parking and less urban congestion, begin at the north end on Route 142. From here the trail is quickly enclosed in a canopy formed by a variety of trees including oak, aspen, maple and cottonwood. Through the trees on your right, you have a bird's-eye view of a suburban neighborhood. On your left rises a wooded hillside that forms a forest backdrop for virtually the length of the path, except where the trail crosses roads. Enjoy this verdant interlude, but don't forget to

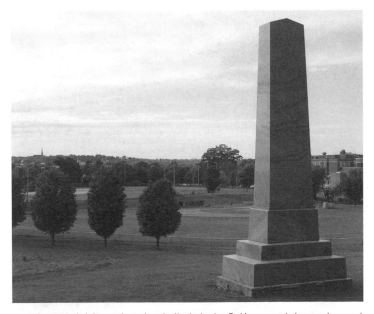

A granite obelisk near the trail marks Knickerbocker Park's memorial playgrounds, a good spot for taking a break to enjoy a view of the valley beyond.

Location
Rensselaer County

Endpoints
Northern Drive
(State Route 142) to
Middleburgh Street
in Troy

Mileage
3.1

Roughness Index
1

Surface
Asphalt

135

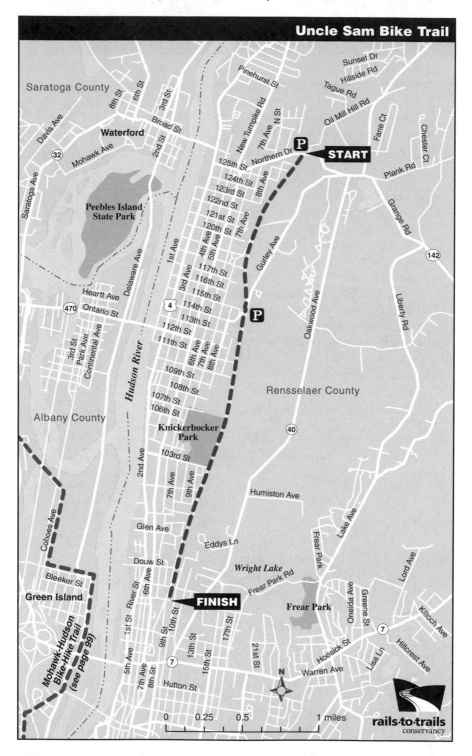

Uncle Sam Bike Trail

Saratoga County

Waterford

32

Davis Ave

Saratoga Ave

Mohawk Ave

8th St

6th St

3rd St

Broad St

2nd St

Pinehurst St

New Turnpike Rd

7th Ave N St

Northern Dr

P

START

Sunset Dr

Hillside Rd

Tague Rd

Oil Mill Hill Rd

Fane Ct

Chester Ct

Plank Rd

Grange Rd

142

125th St

124th St

123rd St

122nd St

121st St

120th St

8th Ave

7th Ave

4th Ave

5th Ave

Peebles Island
State Park

1st Ave

Delaware Ave

Gurley Ave

117th St

116th St

115th St

114th St

113th St

112th St

111th St

3rd Ave

P

Oakwood Ave

Liberty Rd

Heartt Ave

470

Ontario St

4

6th Ave

7th Ave

8th Ave

109th St

108th St

107th St

106th St

Hudson River

3rd St

Park Ave

Continental Ave

Rensselaer County

40

Albany County

2nd Ave

Knickerbocker
Park

103rd St

7th Ave

9th Ave

Humiston Ave

Lake Ave

Cohoes Ave

Glen Ave

Eddys Ln

Wright Lake

Frear Park Rd

Frear Park

Lord Ave

Bleeker St

Green Island

Douw St

6th Ave

1st St

River St

5th St

FINISH

Oneida Ave

Greene St

7

Killoch Ave

Mohawk-Hudson
Bike-Hike Trail
(see page 99)

9th St

10th St

13th St

15th St

17th St

21st St

Hoosick St

Warren Ave

Lisa Ln

Hillcrest Ave

5th Ave

7th Ave

8th Ave

Hutton St

7

N

0   0.25   0.5   1 miles

rails·to·trails
conservancy

watch the trail—it is considerably eroded in some places, and farther south the pavement is occasionally uneven.

About halfway your glimpses of Troy become more urban. At mile 1.7 you pass the buildings and athletic field of the large Lansingburgh High School. A granite obelisk near the trail marks Knickerbocker Park's memorial playgrounds, a good spot for taking a break to enjoy the sweeping view of the valley beyond.

The Uncle Sam Trail follows the corridor of the Boston & Maine Railroad. The B&M brought passenger traffic and a lesser amount of freight traffic to Troy, where travelers could connect with the New York Central and the Delaware & Hudson Railway. Troy was also home to Samuel Wilson, who supplied upstate New York troops with meat during the War of 1812. The story goes that provisions came in barrels stamped "U.S." and soldiers joked that it stood for "Uncle Sam." The name came to stand for the patriotic caricature of the U.S.

At the trail's southern end, you'll emerge from the woods into the city. There is no parking access here and bicyclists take note: Keep your eyes open for broken glass on the trail's last block.

DIRECTIONS

The northern trailhead is in north Troy on State Route 142 (Northern Drive), one block east of 9th Avenue. Look for the trail and parking area on the south side of the highway.

Contact: City of Troy Parks and Recreation
191 103rd Street and 8th Avenue
Troy, NY 12180
(518) 235-7761
http://troyny.gov/recreation/unclesambikeway.html

Walkway Over the Hudson

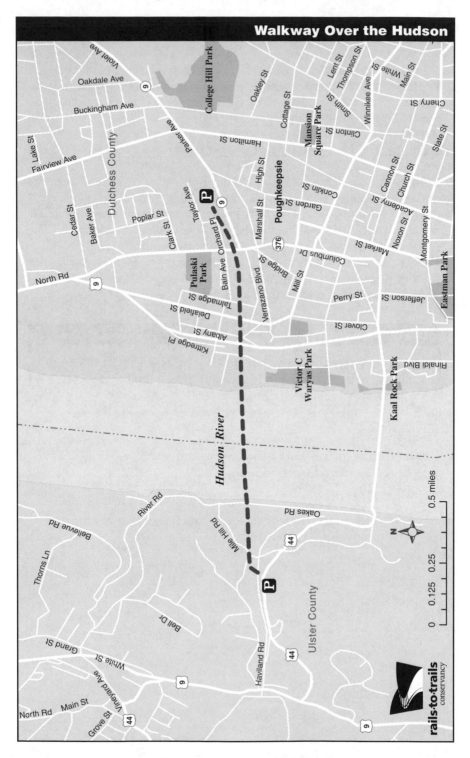

Walkway Over the Hudson

B uilt in 1888 to link New York and New England to the coal beds of Pennsylvania and the West, the steel-truss Poughkeepsie-Highland Railroad Bridge was the longest bridge in the world for a spell, stretching 6,767 feet (approximately 1.25 miles) over the Hudson River. A 1974 blaze, blamed on sparks from a passing train, damaged only 700 feet of the span's wooden decking. Repair, however, was too pricey for the bankrupt railroad company that owned the structure, and tearing it down would have been far more expensive. Instead they permanently halted railroad operations on it.

Today the bridge is the Walkway Over the Hudson State Historic Park. The bridge deck is 212 feet above the Hudson River and provides spectacular views both upstream and down. Expanding 24 feet over land to 35 feet over the water, the deck used to fit a pair of railroad tracks. Now it sees a steady flow of walkers, joggers, skaters and bicyclists who drink in this new view, which opened to the public in late 2009.

Location
Dutchess and Ulster counties

Endpoints
Poughkeepsie to Highland

Mileage
1.25

Roughness Index
1

Surface
Concrete

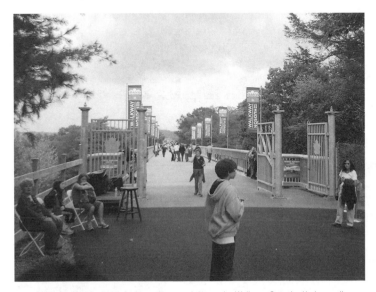

With spectacular views both upstream and down, the Walkway Over the Hudson will one day be a linchpin in a 27-mile corridor of rail-trails and riverfront parks.

It will one day be a linchpin in a 27-mile corridor of rail-trails and riverfront parks already built or planned in Ulster and Dutchess counties. The Hudson Valley Rail Trail's (see page 85) final mile in Highland connects to the bridge's east end. In Poughkeepsie, the Dutchess Rail Trail Park will eventually connect to the bridge at Parker Avenue.

Walkway Over the Hudson started with a group of like-minded locals. In 1992 they formed an advocacy organization devoted to converting the bridge into a public walkway. About 15 years later, they had funding in place and the state was on board to manage and maintain the park. Construction was a considerable undertaking. The entire structure, including underwater piers, had to be assessed for stability. Existing railroad structures such as walkways, ties and railings, were demolished to make way for the new deck's pre-cast concrete panels. Additional metal and foundation repairs were required to support the weight of the crane that would place the panels. Worker safety was a primary concern. Anyone working within 6 feet of the edge was required to wear a harness and lifeline. Select workers with climbing skills were identified as emergency responders in case of a problem.

No skateboards or motorized vehicles are allowed. Pets must be on a leash no longer than 6 feet. Restrooms are available at either end of the bridge.

DIRECTIONS

To reach the trailhead in Poughkeepsie, from Interstate 84, take the Taconic State Parkway north. Exit on State Route 55 west toward Poughkeepsie. Turn right onto Garden Street. Turn left onto Parker Avenue. Parking for the walkway is on the right.

To reach the trailhead in Lloyd, from Interstate 87 take the exit for State Route 299 east. Turn right onto US Route 9W south through the village of Highland. Turn left onto Haviland Road. Parking is on the right.

Contact: Walkway Over the Hudson
P.O. Box 889
Poughkeepsie, NY 12602
(845) 454-9649
http://walkway.org

Wallkill Valley Rail Trail

T he 15-mile Wallkill Valley Rail Trail uses the old Wallkill Valley Railroad bed and extends from Rosendale at Route 213 through its halfway point in New Paltz to the Gardiner and Shawangunk town line. Since much of the corridor north of Rosendale has been acquired, you may someday be able to travel all the way to Kingston.

To conquer the trail in one trip, have a friend drop you off at the northern access point near Route 213 in Rosendale. From Route 213 take Keaton Avenue south, and after crossing the bridge, take the first right as the road starts to climb steeply. In two blocks you come to the beginning of the trail, where Keaton Avenue becomes Mountain Road. Unfortunately at this time you cannot access the 940-foot trestle over Rondout Creek.

When the trail crosses Mountain Road, its surface becomes a mixture of gravel, cinders, grass and dirt. The surrounding landscape is equally mixed. The trail cuts through hillsides, wetlands, forests and fields.

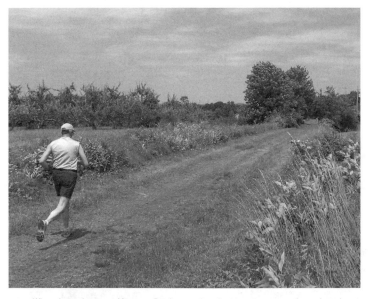

When the trail crosses Mountain Road, its surface becomes a mixture of gravel, cinders, grass and dirt.

Location
Ulster County

Endpoints
High Bridge in Rosendale to Denniston Road at the Gardiner and Shawangunk town line

Mileage
15.2

Roughness Index
2

Surface
Asphalt, ballast, dirt, crushed stone, grass and gravel

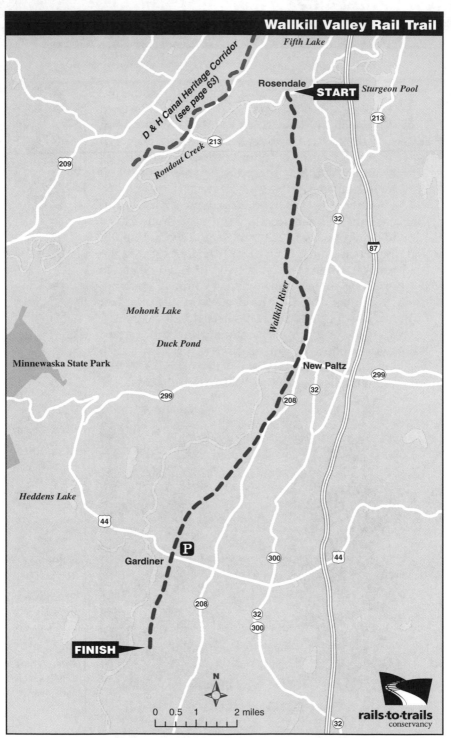

Wallkill Valley Rail Trail

Fifth Lake

Rosendale **START** *Sturgeon Pool*

213

209

213

Rondout Creek

D & H Canal Heritage Corridor
(see page 63)

32

87

Wallkill River

Mohonk Lake

Duck Pond

Minnewaska State Park

New Paltz

299

299

32

208

Heddens Lake

44

P

Gardiner

300

44

208

32

300

FINISH

N

0   0.5   1   2 miles

32

rails·to·trails
conservancy

At about mile 3 you cross Springtown Road, followed by a fine example of a steel-truss bridge over placid Wallkill River. South of the bridge, a viewing platform with benches off of the trail encourages enjoyment of the wetland wildlife. For almost a quarter mile between Plains Road and Broadhead Avenue in New Paltz, the trail is asphalt.

In New Paltz, the trail is adjacent to Huguenot Street, a National Historic Landmark District. At the intersection of the trail and Main Street in New Paltz, a great restaurant occupies the restored former train station. There are shops and additional eateries in New Paltz to tempt the trail user.

South of New Paltz, the trail surface returns to gravel and is a little rougher, but before you leave the outskirts of New Paltz, the trail gives you direct access to the Wallkill. The thick tree stand and cool water offer a refreshing dip on a hot summer day. Much of the next 5 miles pass through agricultural landscape and wetlands. The hedges lining the trail can grow high and thick, but every now and then a view of a small farm or field opens up. The trail ends suddenly at Denniston Road at the Gardiner and Shawangunk town line, but it's more convenient to load bikes in the hamlet of Gardiner, which has parking and an excellent ice cream shop on the trail as well.

DIRECTIONS

To reach the Rosendale endpoint, take the New Paltz exit off Interstate 87 (New York State Thruway). Turn left on State Route 299/Main Street. Turn right on State Route 32. Stay on Route 32 when it merges with State Route 213. Turn left on Tilson Road. Turn right onto Springtown Road. Springtown Road becomes Elting Road. Turn left onto Mountain Road. The trail begins just before you reach Fairview Avenue.

To reach the Gardiner trailhead, take the New Paltz exit off Interstate 87 (New York State Thruway). Turn left on State Route 299/Main Street. New New Paltz, turn left on to State Route 208. Follow this to the intersection of Highway 44/State Route 55, and turn right. Now on Main Street head west into downtown Gardiner, then turn right on 2nd Street. Parking is on the left.

Contact: Wallkill Valley Rail Trail Association
P.O. Box 1048
New Paltz, NY 12561
www.gorailtrail.org

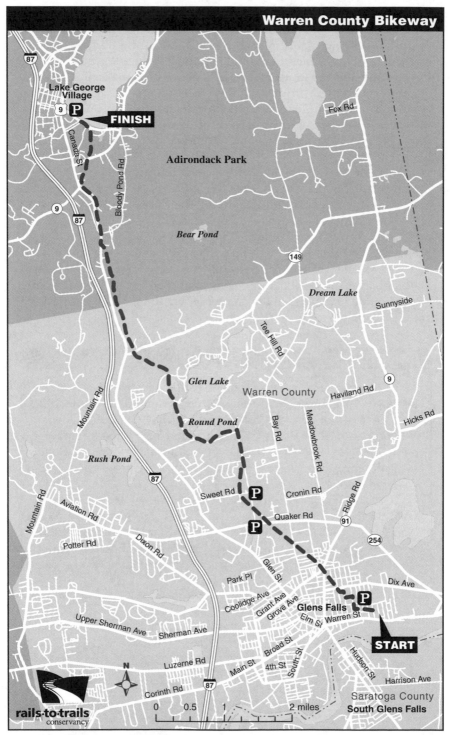

Warren County Bikeway

Lake George Village

FINISH

Adirondack Park

Fox Rd

Canada St

Bloody Pond Rd

Bear Pond

149

Dream Lake

Sunnyside

Tee Hill Rd

Glen Lake

Warren County

Haviland Rd

Mountain Rd

Round Pond

Bay Rd

Meadowbrook Rd

Hicks Rd

Rush Pond

87

Sweet Rd

Cronin Rd

Ridge Rd

91

Aviation Rd

Quaker Rd

254

Mountain Rd

Dixon Rd

Potter Rd

Park Pl

Glen St

Dix Ave

Coolidge Ave

Grant Ave

Grove Ave

Glens Falls

START

Upper Sherman Ave

Sherman Ave

Elm St

Warren St

Luzerne Rd

Main St

4th St

Broad St

South St

Hudson St

Harrison Ave

Corinth Rd

87

Saratoga County

South Glens Falls

N

0   0.5   1   2 miles

rails·to·trails
conservancy

Warren County Bikeway

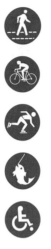

T his trail is as smart as it is pretty. Signs that detail the area's history and appealing destinations accompany a scenic ride from Glens Falls into the resort town of Lake George, New York. Traveling by bicycle in either direction, you can stretch your legs with some climbing. Begin in Glens Falls to take advantage of a more gradual ascent and the reward of a swim at Lake George Beach.

The trail's south end at Platt Street does not have designated parking, so leave your car at the Leonard Street Trailhead. Then, to say you rode the entire trail, follow the bikeway signs south on Leonard Street a couple of blocks watching for where the trail picks up on your left.

You will see several 19th-century industrial buildings along the trail, and the tracks of the Delaware and Hudson Railway (D&H) are visible on the far side of Platt Street. The D & H took passengers all the way from New York City through Glens Falls to the resort town

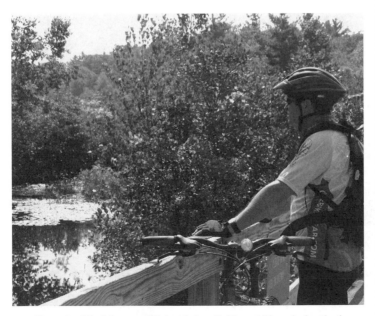

The tracks of the Delaware and Hudson Railway (D&H) are visible on the far side of Platt Street.

Location
Warren County

Endpoints
Platt Street in Glens Falls to Lake George Beach State Park in Lake George Village

Mileage
10

Roughness Index
1

Surface
Asphalt

145

then known as Caldwell (now Lake George). Today much of the bike path follows that route.

Return to the Leonard Street Trailhead and follow the trail, heading west and north through a residential and light industrial area. Less than a mile ahead, the trailside Coopers Cave Ale Company has a bike rack and picnic tables if you hanker for a gourmet soda or handmade ice cream. As you near Queensbury, trees green the trail, and at mile 2.2 you cross the beautiful pedestrian bridge over Quaker Road and Halfway Brook. After another trailside ice cream opportunity, at Sprinkles, the trail becomes wooded. You just might see a fox cross the trail.

At about mile 3.3 you will leave the trail for 1.5 miles. The well-marked detour takes roads past large homes and the Glens Falls Country Club. The surroundings become more forested as you return to the bike trail. Then views of glittery Glen Lake, considered an idyllic fishing spot, reward your climbing efforts. As you cross a bridge over the lake's feeder stream you will probably spy aquatic wildlife, water lilies, and other flowering water plants.

Until you reach Route 149, about 1.2 miles north, you follow the right-of-way of the old Hudson Valley Railway, which provided trolley and interurban services. Woods and meadows again surround you; a stream gurgles beside the trail, which trends uphill.

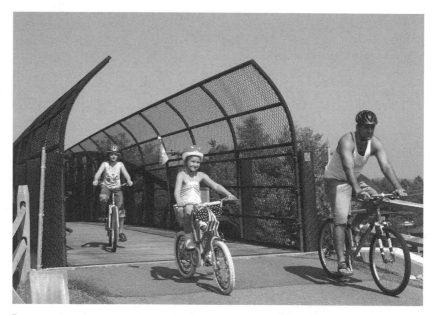

Trees green the trail as you cross the beautiful pedestrian bridge over Quaker Road and Halfway Brook.

At mile 8 the trail briefly parallels busy Route 9, and you will see the 30-foot *Uncle Sam* statue in the Magic Forest theme park. From here it's all downhill to Lake George Village, rife with sites cultural and historical, such as the Spanish Mission–style train station. As the trail winds down at the shore of the beautiful lake, it cuts through Lake George Beach State Park. Don't forget that swim!

DIRECTIONS

To reach the Glens Falls Trailhead, take Interstate 87 to Exit 18, then head east on the combination Corinth Road and Broad Street for about a mile. Bear left on South Street. Cross Glen Street (Route 9), where South becomes Bay Street. Go one block, then turn right on Maple Street. After several blocks, turn left on Leonard Street. Go 1½ blocks and look for the trailhead and parking on the left.

To reach the Lake George Beach Trailhead, take Interstate 87 to Exit 21, and take Route 9 North. Turn left at the traffic light, continuing on Route 9. In less than a mile, at the bottom of the hill on Route 9, bear right, following a sign for Lake George Beach. Head up this road and park alongside it. The trail begins at the end of the road on your right next to a signboard.

Contact: Warren County Parks and Recreation Department
Parks and Recreation Office
Warren County Fish Hatchery
145 Echo Lake Road
Warrensburg, NY 12885
(518) 623-2877
www.warrencountydpw.com

Warren County Tourism Office
1340 State Route 9
Warren County Municipal Center
Lake George, NY 12845
(518) 761-6366
www.visitlakegeorge.com

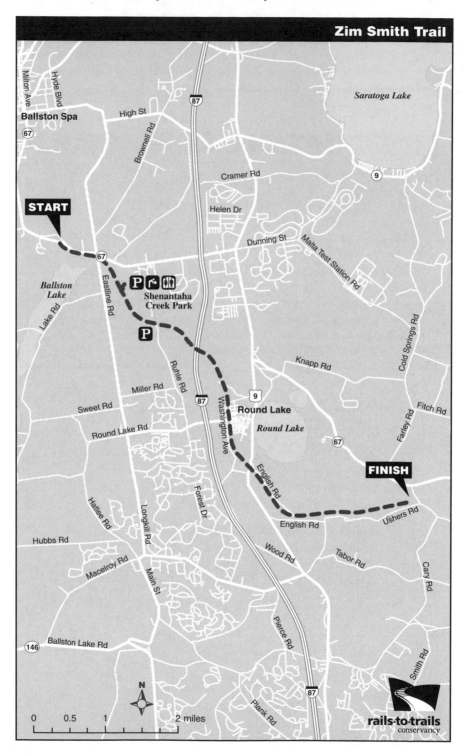

Zim Smith Trail

Saratoga Lake

Milton Ave

Hyde Blvd

Ballston Spa
67

High St

Brownell Rd

87

9

Cramer Rd

Helen Dr

START

Dunning St

Malta Test Station Rd

67

Eastline Rd

Ballston
Lake

P 🚶 🚻
Shenantaha
Creek Park

P

Lake Rd

Cold Springs Rd

Ruhle Rd

Miller Rd

Knapp Rd

87

Sweet Rd

9

Round Lake

Round Lake Rd

Round Lake

Washington Ave

67

Fitch Rd

Farley Rd

FINISH

Hallee Rd

Longkill Rd

Forest Dr

English Rd

English Rd

Ushers Rd

Hubbs Rd

Macelroy Rd

Main St

Wood Rd

Tabor Rd

Cary Rd

146
Ballston Lake Rd

N

Smith Rd

Pierce Rd

87

0   0.5   1   2 miles

Plank Rd

rails·to·trails
conservancy

Zim Smith Trail

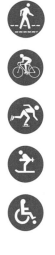

The Zim Smith Trail, sometimes called the Zim Smith Mid-County Trail, connects the town of Halfmoon with Round Lake Village, Clifton Park, Malta and Ballston. A 1.75-mile extension to Ballston Spa was completed in October 2010.

The best place to start is at Malta's Shenantaha Creek Park, about 2.75 miles south of the northern terminus. The park offers convenient access to the rail-trail and is an appealing destination in its own right. The park's picnic tables, playground equipment, tennis courts and volleyball net could turn an exercise session into a full afternoon's outing.

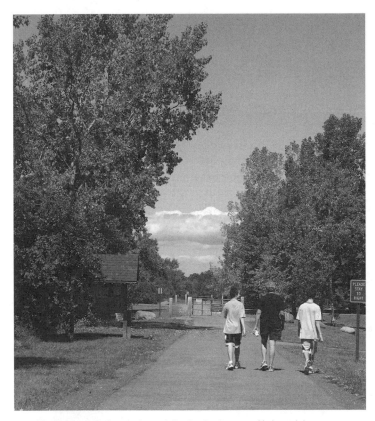

The Zim Smith Trail is mostly wooded with a few homes visible beyond the trees as you leave the park.

Location
Saratoga County

Endpoints
Overpass Road
in Malta to Coons
Crossing Road
in Halfmoon

Mileage
6

**Roughness
Index**
1

Surface
Asphalt and
crushed stone

As you enter the trail from the parking lot, turn left to head toward the Village of Round Lake and Halfmoon. The rail-trail is, for the most part, wooded with a few homes visible beyond the trees as you leave the park. The trail rolls gently downhill, with pretty views into a ravine to your left, and a slope rising to your right.

About a mile south of the park, the trail passes under Interstate 87, or the Adirondack Northway. Nearing Round Lake, the trail is more settled, and you can see backyards and horse pastures through the trees.

A handsome white frame church, other period buildings and a welcome sign signal your arrival in Round Lake Village. Treat yourself to a spin around the quiet streets of this Victorian hamlet and its ornate "gingerbread cottages." The village was a Methodist camp meeting site that swelled with thousands of visitors each summer. The 1885 Round Lake Auditorium, at 7th and Wesley streets, is home to a 34-foot-tall, historically significant pipe organ. The auditorium is still in use—not for delivering sermons, but with a lively performing arts program.

From Round Lake Village the trail crosses over Route 9 and through a portion of Town of Clifton Park. The trail turns east upon leaving the park. A pond on the south side of the trail signals the end of the developed trail at Coons Crossing Road.

DIRECTIONS

To reach the Shenantaha Creek Park Trailhead in Malta, from Interstate 87, take Exit 12 to the traffic circle and head west on Route 67. Continue on Route 67 until it intersects East Line Road at a traffic light. Turn left on East Line Road and go about 0.5 mile, watching for the park entrance on your left. Follow the entrance road to the parking lot and trail.

Contact: Saratoga County
50 West High Street
Ballston Spa, NY 12020
(518) 884-4705
www.saratogacountyny.gov

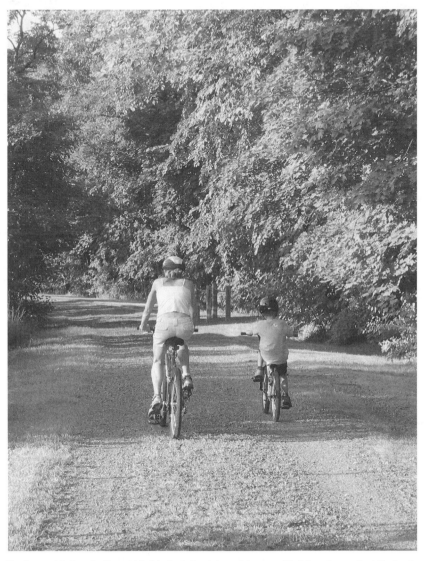

The Raymond G. Esposito Memorial Trail in South Nyack is a milelong gravel trail through several neighborhoods on the Hudson River. From its start in a community park, the rail-trail heads south, occasionally high above some of the neighborhoods it passes.

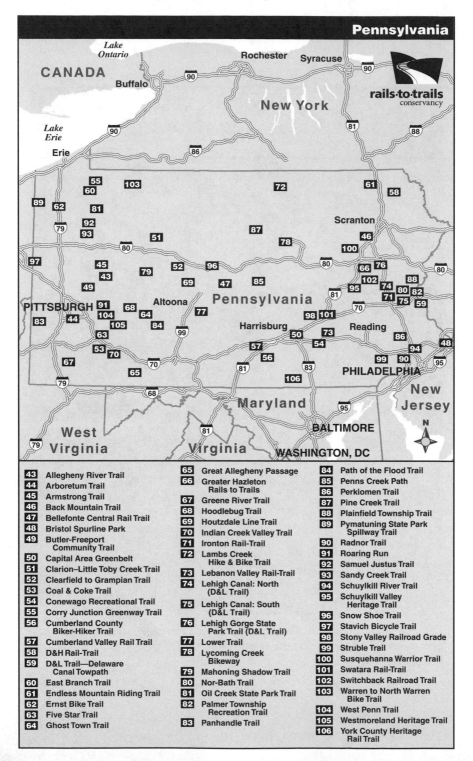

Pennsylvania

Lake Ontario

Rochester Syracuse

CANADA

Buffalo

rails·to·trails
conservancy

New York

Lake Erie

Erie

Scranton

PITTSBURGH Altoona **Pennsylvania**

Harrisburg Reading

PHILADELPHIA

West Virginia

Virginia

Maryland

BALTIMORE

WASHINGTON, DC

New Jersey

43	Allegheny River Trail
44	Arboretum Trail
45	Armstrong Trail
46	Back Mountain Trail
47	Bellefonte Central Rail Trail
48	Bristol Spurline Park
49	Butler-Freeport Community Trail
50	Capital Area Greenbelt
51	Clarion–Little Toby Creek Trail
52	Clearfield to Grampian Trail
53	Coal & Coke Trail
54	Conewago Recreational Trail
55	Corry Junction Greenway Trail
56	Cumberland County Biker-Hiker Trail
57	Cumberland Valley Rail Trail
58	D&H Rail-Trail
59	D&L Trail—Delaware Canal Towpath
60	East Branch Trail
61	Endless Mountain Riding Trail
62	Ernst Bike Trail
63	Five Star Trail
64	Ghost Town Trail

65	Great Allegheny Passage
66	Greater Hazleton Rails to Trails
67	Greene River Trail
68	Hoodlebug Trail
69	Houtzdale Line Trail
70	Indian Creek Valley Trail
71	Ironton Rail-Trail
72	Lambs Creek Hike & Bike Trail
73	Lebanon Valley Rail-Trail
74	Lehigh Canal: North (D&L Trail)
75	Lehigh Canal: South (D&L Trail)
76	Lehigh Gorge State Park Trail (D&L Trail)
77	Lower Trail
78	Lycoming Creek Bikeway
79	Mahoning Shadow Trail
80	Nor-Bath Trail
81	Oil Creek State Park Trail
82	Palmer Township Recreation Trail
83	Panhandle Trail

84	Path of the Flood Trail
85	Penns Creek Path
86	Perkiomen Trail
87	Pine Creek Trail
88	Plainfield Township Trail
89	Pymatuning State Park Spillway Trail
90	Radnor Trail
91	Roaring Run
92	Samuel Justus Trail
93	Sandy Creek Trail
94	Schuylkill River Trail
95	Schuylkill Valley Heritage Trail
96	Snow Shoe Trail
97	Stavich Bicycle Trail
98	Stony Valley Railroad Grade
99	Struble Trail
100	Susquehanna Warrior Trail
101	Swatara Rail-Trail
102	Switchback Railroad Trail
103	Warren to North Warren Bike Trail
104	West Penn Trail
105	Westmoreland Heritage Trail
106	York County Heritage Rail Trail

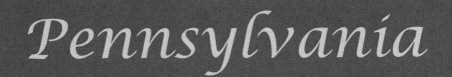

Pennsylvania

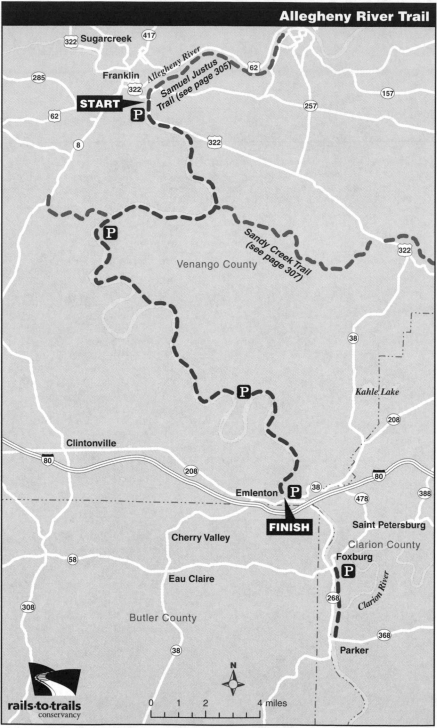

Allegheny River Trail

322 Sugarcreek 417

285

Franklin
Allegheny River
62
322
Samuel Justus Trail (see page 305)

START
P

62

8

257

157

322

P

Venango County

Sandy Creek Trail (see page 307)

322

38

Kahle Lake

208

P

Clintonville

80

208

Emlenton P
38
80

478
388

FINISH

Saint Petersburg

Cherry Valley

Clarion County

58

Foxburg
P

Eau Claire

268

Clarion River

308

Butler County

38

368

Parker

N

rails·to·trails
conservancy

0 1 2 4 miles

Allegheny River Trail

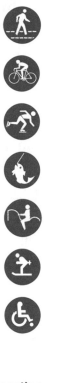

With a wide, paved pathway and adjacent equestrian trail running through lush woodland and riverside terrain, the Allegheny River Trail (ART) has something to offer every trail enthusiast. Following a segment of the Allegheny River that is part of the National Wild and Scenic Rivers System, the 32-mile trail extends south from the Samuel Justus Trail (see page 305) in Franklin, to the point where the Allegheny and Clarion rivers meet in Brandon.

The Scrubgrass Generating Company acquired the rail corridor after the Allegheny Valley Railroad stopped using it in 1984. Scrubgrass Generating turned around and donated the property to the nonprofit Allegheny Valley Trails Association, which is building an extensive rail-trail system in northwestern Pennsylvania.

The trailhead begins 5 miles downriver from the Franklin Belmar railroad bridge. Built in 1907 the

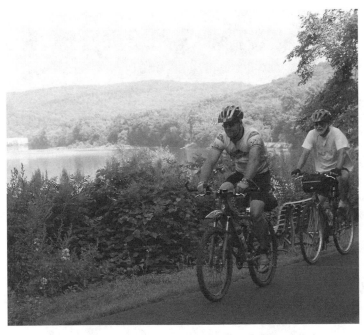

The views of the river and wildlife from the Allegheny River Trail are spectacular.

Location
Clarion and
Venango counties

Endpoints
Franklin to Brandon

Mileage
32

Roughness Index
1

Surface
Paved

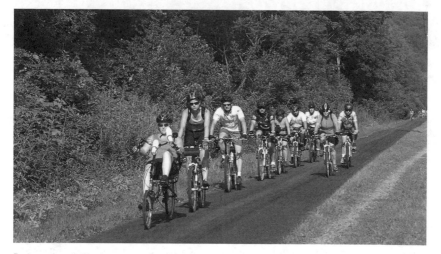

From a wide, paved pathway to an adjacent equestrian trail running through lush woodland and riverside terrain, this trail has something to offer every enthusiast.

picturesque bridge offers a spectacular view of the river and wildlife. At the Belmar bridge, the trail connects with the 8-mile, paved Sandy Creek Trail, that runs east to the village of Van. Eventually it will connect with the Clarion Highlands Trail to offer 46 miles of trail.

DIRECTIONS

To reach the Franklin Trailhead, take Route 8 North to its junction with US 322. Take US 322, which becomes 8th Street in Franklin and crosses the Allegheny River. The trailhead parking lot is on the right. The lot sign says SAMUEL JUSTUS TRAIL, which is the rail-trail going north from Franklin. The Allegheny Trail goes south from the lot.

To reach the Belmar Trailhead for both the Allegheny River and Sandy Creek trails, take Route 8 South from Franklin. Continue 3 miles, turn left on Pone Lane, and pass Sandy Creek High School. Continue to Belmar Road. Turn right on Belmar, and follow the road to the trailhead parking lot at the river.

Contact: Allegheny Valley Trails Association
Box 264
Franklin, PA 16323
(814) 432-4476
www.avta-trails.org

Arboretum Trail

A shining example of what dedicated volunteers can accomplish, the Arboretum Trail is also one of Pennsylvania's twelve rails-with-trails, where trains and trail users share a corridor. Conceived by the Garden Club of Oakmont in 1989 as a centennial gift to the community, the milelong pedestrian-only Arboretum Trail is part of Oakmont's Boulevard Project, an ambitious plan for renovation of a downtown business corridor. An oasis of green and growing beauty and a tangible asset to its community, the Arboretum Trail is a delightful year-round stroll down the lovely landscaped trail through downtown Oakmont.

The rail corridor has a dramatic history of use—and disuse. Between 1853 and 1856, the Allegheny Valley Railroad built a line that ran from Pittsburgh to Kittanning, and passed through the heart of Oakmont Borough. In 1903, the Pennsylvania Railroad opened its Brilliant Cutoff, linking the Allegheny River line with

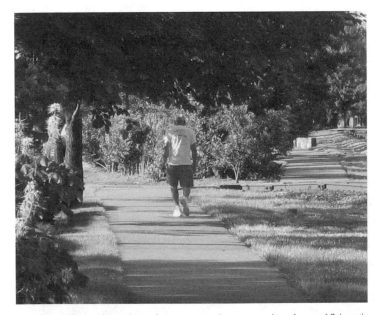

This milelong trail gets plenty of use, no matter the season, and is a feature of Oakmont's downtown revitalization.

Location
Allegheny County

Endpoints
Hulton Road to Plum Street in Oakmont

Mileage
1.4

Roughness Index
1

Surface
Asphalt

157

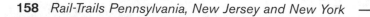

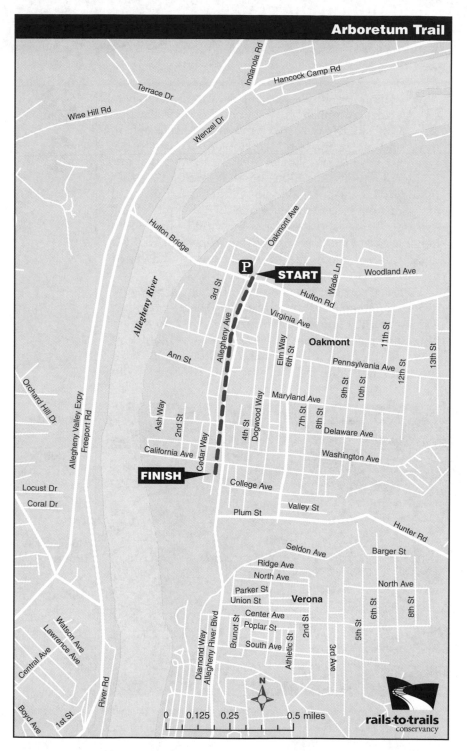

other sections of the city and greatly improving rail service in the area. But declining rail traffic in the 1960s led then-owner Conrail to close one of the two tracks in the borough; during the 1970s the inactive track was removed. Then in 1995, the corridor was sold back to the Allegheny Valley Railroad, which reopened the line and sold the adjacent corridor for trail development

The Garden Club raised $3 million for trail construction, landscaping, corridor renovation and long-term maintenance of the plantings.

DIRECTIONS

From the Pennsylvania Turnpike, take Exit 48 for Allegheny Valley and bear right past the toll booth. Follow the signs to Oakmont and, about a mile from the exit, cross the Hulton Bridge. To find a parking space, turn right just before or after the railroad crossing on Hulton Road onto either Allegheny Avenue or Allegheny River Boulevard. The trail runs between the two streets.

From downtown Pittsburgh, take Route 28 north to the Blawnox exit. Continue along Freeport Road, then turn right onto the Hulton Bridge. Park anywhere along Allegheny Avenue just west of the corridor.

Contact: Oakmont Borough Manager
Oakmont Municipal Building
5th and Virginia Avenue
Oakmont, PA 15139
(412) 828-3232
www.oakmont-pa.com/gov.cfm

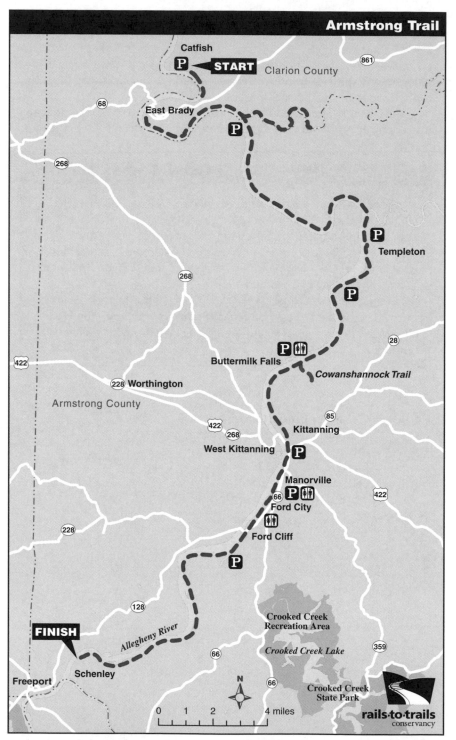

Armstrong Trail

Tracing the course of the scenic Allegheny River, the Armstrong Trail varies between rough terrain and smooth asphalt surfaces to accommodate cyclists, pedestrians, inline skaters and equestrians in the warmer months. There are plenty of opportunities to take photographs of the lazy Allegheny River, and even try your luck catching fish. Cross-country skiers can enjoy the trail in winter.

The Armstrong Trail runs along the former Allegheny Valley Railroad. The railroad, chartered in 1837, and opened in 1855 served as a passenger and freight rail line and eventually extended from Pittsburgh, Pennsylvania, to Buffalo, New York. The rail line ended passenger operations in 1941 and was purchased by the Allegheny Valley Land Trust in 1992 for conversion to the existing trail.

The winding trail extends almost 35 miles, from Catfish on the north end southward to Schenley. The uppermost segment, north of Templeton, features

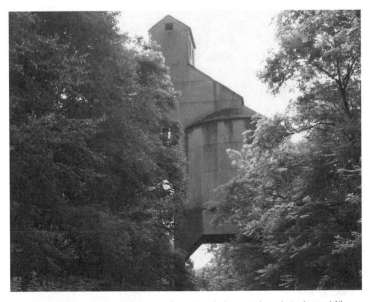

A gigantic concrete coal elevator used to replenish the engine's coal supplies and fill freight cars can be seen along the Armstrong Trail.

Location
Armstrong and Clarion counties

Endpoints
Catfish to Schenley

Mileage
34.8

Roughness Index
3

Surface
Ballast, dirt, grass and asphalt

rough terrain, best suited for mountain biking and hiking. You may encounter the occasional ATV riders or equestrians here too. Relics of the original rail line, including a gigantic concrete coal elevator used to replenish the engine's coal supplies as well as fill freight cars, can be seen along this part of the trail. The section south of Rosston features a similar surface and excitement.

Between Templeton and Rosston, the trail alternates between asphalt path and quiet on-road sections. The town of Kittanning, just south of the trail midpoint, makes for a nice rest stop, with local shops and eateries not far off the trail. Several locks, managed by the Army Corps of Engineers are visible along the trail; you may be lucky enough to see a boat or barge passing through one.

The best access points north of Kittanning at Buttermilk Falls and in Templeton. The parking area at Buttermilk Falls also provides access to the Cowanshannock Trail, a short 1.5-mile rail-trail.

The trail runs close to a number of private residences at many points along the entire trail, so please respect any posted no-trespassing signs. The trail is wheelchair-accessible within the town of Kittanning. The Kiski-Junction Railroad has reactivated an 8-mile section of the rail corridor north of Schenley. Please refer to the trail's website for updates on best access to the trail in this area.

DIRECTIONS

To reach the midpoint at the Buttermilk Falls Trailhead, follow Johnston Avenue north out of Kittaning. Continue north until McMillen Road. Immediately after McMillen, turn right into the parking lot for the Bernard C. Snyder Picnic Area. The Armstrong Trailhead is on the other side of Johnston Ave.

To reach the Templeton Trailhead, travel north on Route 28 from Kittanning. Turn left onto Ridge Road, and left again onto State Route 1034. Turn right onto State Route 1031 (Mosgrove-Templeton Road), and left to continue on 1031. Follow 1031 into the town of Templeton. Turn left on 1st Street, and right on Allegheny Avenue. Park by the boat ramps on the left next to the Allegheny River. The trailhead is accessed next to Allegheny Avenue.

Contact: Allegheny Valley Land Trust
P.O. Box 777
Kittanning, PA 16201
(724) 543-4478
www.armstrongtrail.org

Back Mountain Trail

The Back Mountain Trail, originally built by lumber and ice king Albert Lewis of Wyoming Valley 115 years ago, was acquired by the Lehigh Valley Railroad in 1887. Lumber, ice, leather goods and anthracite coal were milled, tanned, mined and routed to urban markets and steel mills from the Endless Mountains and Susquehanna River Basin well into the 1940s. The corridor fell into disuse in 1963.

In 1996, Anthracite Scenic Trails Association acquired easements and recorded deeds with Luzerne County for public use of the corridor. Eventually, 14 miles will be developed from Riverfront Park on the Susquehanna River in Wilkes-Barre to Harvey's Lake, bringing back memories and supporting a new mode of travel in the region.

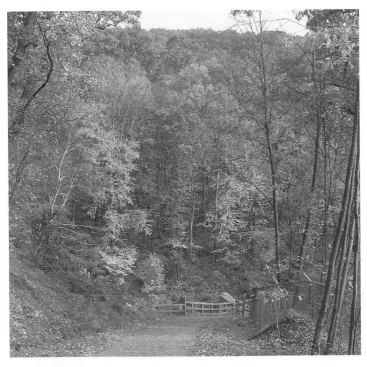

The 4.5-mile Back Mountain Trail is set in scenic woodlands.

Location
Luzerne County

Endpoints
Parry Street in Luzerne to Carverton Road in Trucksville

Mileage
4.5

Roughness Index
1

Surface
Crushed stone

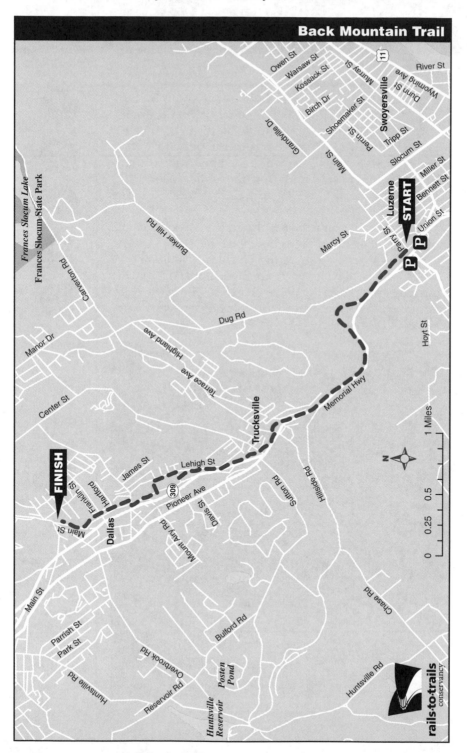

Back Mountain Trail

Today you'll find a 4.5-mile trail that cuts through scenic woodlands complete with a meandering creek, a pretty waterfall and open fields of flowers. Sections of the trail run close to the highway, but don't compromise the feeling of getting away from it all.

DIRECTIONS

To reach the Back Mountain Trail from Interstate 81, take Exit 170 onto State Route 309 North. Take Exit 5/6 and drive north on Main Street to a four-way stop sign. Continue straight ahead onto Parry Street. There's parking at the Knights of Columbus lot. Walk up to the Gateway to the Back Mountain Trailhead.
This trail is wheelchair-accessible.

Contact: Anthracite Scenic Trails Association
P.O. Box 212
Dallas, PA 18612
(570) 675-9016
http://course.wilkes.edu/bmt

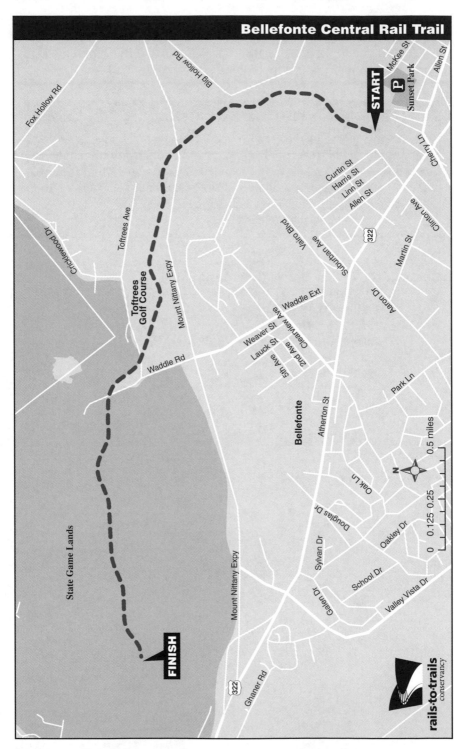

Bellefonte Central Rail Trail

Serene year-round, the Bellefonte Central Rail Trail (BCRT) in central Pennsylvania runs along 1.3 miles of the old Buffalo Run, Bellefonte and Bald Eagle Railroad corridor. The original 19-mile line connecting the towns of Bellefonte and State College, home to Pennsylvania State University, was built in the mid-1880s to move iron ore. It changed hands in 1892 to become the Bellefonte Railroad, and transported passengers, including many students and freight, until it ceased operation in the 1980s. In 1953 President Dwight Eisenhower and First Lady Mamie Eisenhower traveled on the Bellefonte Central to visit Dwight's brother, then-president of Penn State.

The Bellefonte Central Rail Trail is part of the master plan for the Arboretum at Penn State, where it will be a major artery through the site. Visitors and staff will use it to reach the botanical gardens, wetlands and research facilities, and, closer to the trail, woodlands that

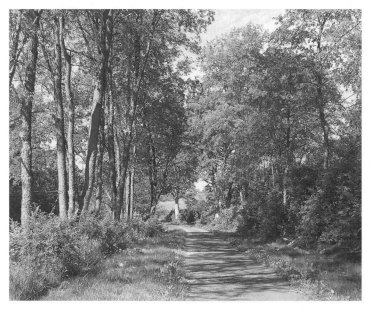

Many Penn State students commute on the Bellefonte Central Rail Trail.

Location
Centre County

Endpoints
McKee Street and Clinton Avenue Bike Path off Sunset Park to Toftrees Avenue

Mileage
1.3

Roughness Index
3

Surface
Stone dust

are being restored to the oak and hickory forest that dominated the area before invasive, nonnative plants appeared.

The trail sets out a quarter mile west of Sunset Park along the McKee Street and Clinton Avenue Bike Path. The southern end of the trail is less than a mile from Pennsylvania State University, making the trail a popular route for commuting students. For most of the way it is tree-lined with open fields beyond the shade-lending serene pastoral views till it ends after passing over a culvert and shortly before reaching the Mt. Nittany Expressway overpass.

An informal trail extends nearly 2 more miles to Toftrees Resort and Golf Course, residential areas and beyond, ending at Montauk Circle in the town of Port Matilda. At its far reaches, the trail becomes rugged and is best suited for pedestrians or mountain bikes. A feasibility study is looking into extending the developed trail to Toftrees and another 13 miles to Bellefonte in the future.

DIRECTIONS

To reach the McKee Street Trailhead from Interstate 80 west, take Exit 161, turn left and follow US 220 South 11 miles toward Bellefonte. Take Exit 74 toward Penn State University on East Park Avenue. At 2.3 miles turn right at McKee Street. At the end of McKee Street (about seven blocks) are Sunset Park (with parking and restroom facilities) on the left and McKee Street and Clinton Avenue Bike Path straight ahead. Follow the bike path downhill less than a quarter mile to the flat where the Bellefonte Central Rail Trail begins.

Contact: The Arboretum at Penn State
Pennsylvania State University
336 Forest Resources Building
University Park, PA 16802
(814) 865-9118
www.arboretum.psu.edu

Bristol Spurline Park

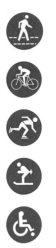

Since it opened as a railroad spur in the 1800s, this pretty trail has always been about connections. In 1834, the Philadelphia and Trenton Railroad launched the spur to carry goods from Bristol, Pennsylvania, then a bustling little port where the Delaware division of the Pennsylvania canal system met the tidewater of the Delaware River.

The canal still exists in Bristol, but the original main line of the Philadelphia and Trenton railroad was relocated in 1882. That line became Amtrak's New York to Washington corridor, one of the most heavily traveled passenger railroad routes in the country. Conrail donated the old spur line to the town of Bristol, and the trail opened in 1980.

The path incorporates the rail corridor and some of the former canal towpath, carrying trail users to the Bristol Marsh, a unique and sensitive freshwater habitat. Traversing downtown Bristol, this residential trail

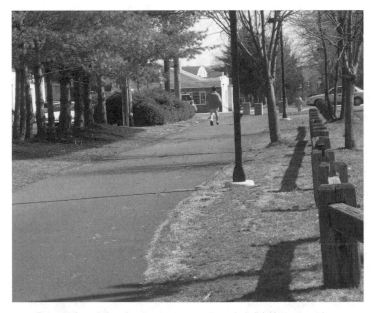

This smooth, asphalt-surfaced trail connects with nearby ball fields, grassy parks, retirement communities and an elementary school.

Location
Bucks County

Endpoints
Mill Street to
Radcliffe Street
in Bristol

Mileage
2.5

**Roughness
Index**
1

Surface
Asphalt

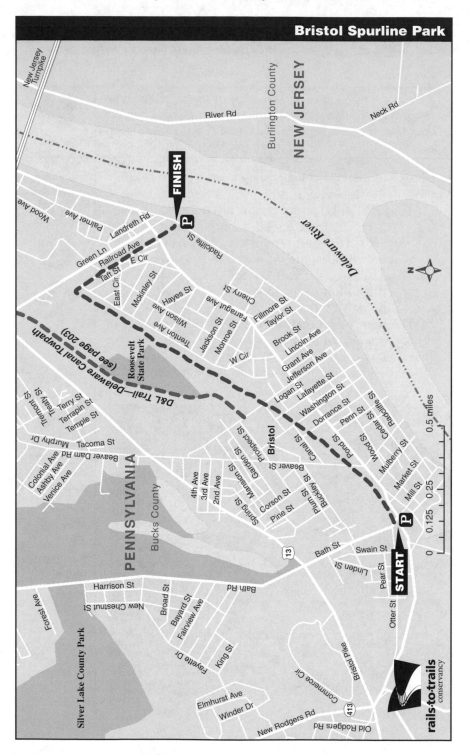

eventually will provide public access to the Delaware River and waterfront at the end of Green Lane. This smooth, asphalt-surfaced trail also connects with nearby ball fields, grassy parks, retirement communities and an elementary school.

DIRECTIONS

From the Pennsylvania Turnpike, take the Bristol exit. Take Green Lane into the Borough of Bristol. Turn right on Radcliffe Street and continue through the historic district to the Bristol Spurline Park parking lot at the end of the street. Trailhead is marked at the parking lot.

This trail is wheelchair-accessible.

Contact: PA State Parks
250 Pond St.
Bristol, PA 19007
(215) 788-3828, extension 10
www.visitpa.com/visitpa/details.pa?id=59704

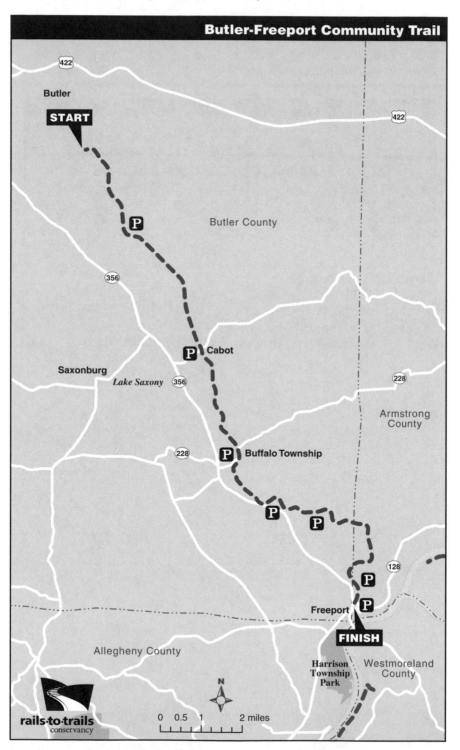

Butler-Freeport Community Trail

422

Butler

START

356

Butler County

422

P

P **Cabot**

Saxonburg

Lake Saxony 356

228

P **Buffalo Township**

228

Armstrong County

P

P

128

P

Freeport P

FINISH

Allegheny County

Harrison Township Park

Westmoreland County

rails·to·trails
conservancy

N

0   0.5   1   2 miles

Butler-Freeport Community Trail

Built in 1871 to transport the region's high-quality limestone to support Pittsburgh's growing steel industry, the Butler-Freeport line was the first railroad in the county. After a two-day celebration of the opening, the railroad conducted a mock funeral for the stagecoach that ran between the two towns. A branch of the Western Pennsylvania Railroad, the line became part of the Pennsylvania Railroad system in 1903 before closing.

The 16-mile Butler-Freeport Community Trail on the corridor, open since 1989, is nestled in the scenic wooded valley that follows Little Buffalo Creek to Buffalo Creek and on to the Allegheny River at Freeport.

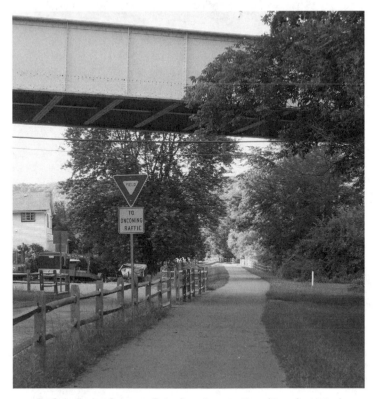

Location
Armstrong and
Butler counties

Endpoints
Butler and Freeport

Mileage
16

Roughness Index
1

Surface
Crushed stone, dirt
and asphalt

The Butler-Freeport Community Trail is flat and easy to ride, and its surface varies from crushed stone to dirt to asphalt.

About an hour northeast of the City of Pittsburgh, the trail is flat and easy to ride. Heading south from Butler, you'll be on a slight incline. The trail surface changes from crushed stone to dirt to asphalt.

Remains of old stone quarries and brick kilns can be seen in the southern section of the trail. Heading north from Cabot, the results of late 1800 development are still visible. The former Saxon City Hotel, built in 1871, remains, as does an old, still active lumberyard.

From April to October you can see an abundance of wildflowers, including trillium, Turk's cap lily, tall bellflower and butterfly weed. The trail is a popular recreation venue. Visitors come to enjoy bird watching and fishing, and the annual fall Buffalo Creek Half-Marathon always attracts a crowd. Before leaving Freeport, stop by the Freeport Area Historical Society office, where you'll find a wealth of information on the cultural and industrial history of the region.

The Butler-Freeport Trail Council maintains a passport-oriented historic geocache adventure with up to 20 caches along the trail. Check their website for details.

DIRECTIONS

To reach the Butler Trailhead, from Pittsburgh, take Route 28 North to a left onto Route 356 North. Go about 4 miles to Sarver Road. Bear right on Sarver Road and go a mile to Buffalo Township Fire Station, which will be on your left. Park in the upper lot at the fire station. This access area is 3 miles from the southern end and 7 miles from the northern end of the trail.

Contact: Butler-Freeport Trail Council
P.O. Box 533
Saxonburg, PA 16056
(724) 352-4783
www.butlerfreeporttrail.org

Capital Area Greenbelt

Originally conceived by landscape architect Warren Manning (a disciple of Frederick Law Olmsted), the Capital Area Greenbelt is a 20-mile ring of parks and trails encircling the Pennsylvania capital city of Harrisburg. In the early 1900s, the greenbelt was partially constructed in accordance with Manning's plan, but the project was never fully realized and much of the greenbelt fell into disuse and disrepair. Since 1991, a group of volunteers, the Capital Area Greenbelt Association, has worked with state and local government, businesses, foundations, and citizens to improve the trail.

Segments of the greenbelt were originally roughed in by volunteers, using grass and wood chips, and have now been converted to a crushed limestone surface or paved. Where necessary, the greenbelt uses signed road routes to connect the trail sections. Volunteers have focused on the park and open space components of the greenbelt and created the Five Senses Garden, a popular waypoint along the trail.

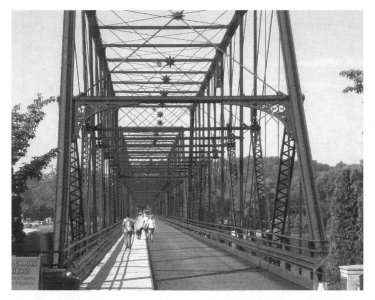

The Walnut Street Bridge, or the "People's Bridge," is a restored iron trestle bridge between City Island and the riverfront walkway along Front Street in Harrisburg.

Location
Dauphin County

Endpoints
City Island in Harrisburg

Mileage
20

Roughness Index
1

Surface
Asphalt and concrete

175

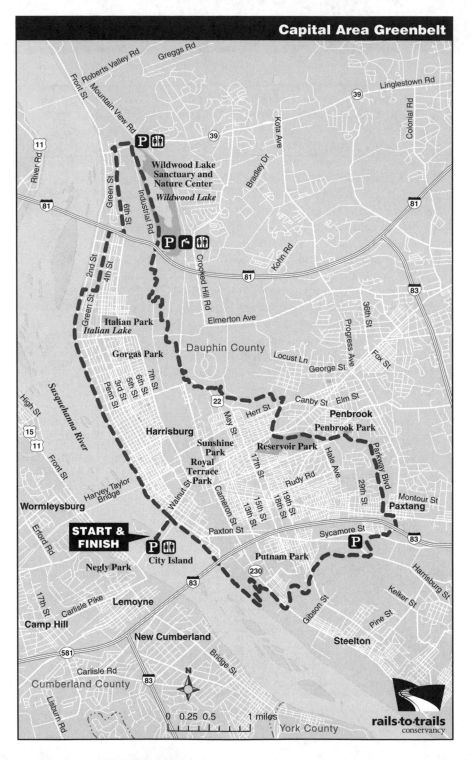

Capital Area Greenbelt

The greenbelt is a loop trail with many access points along its route, but the best parking is on City Island in Harrisburg, a popular multiuse recreational destination in the middle of the Susquehanna River.

At the northern edge of the city lies another popular starting point or destination along the trail. Wildwood Lake Sanctuary and Nature Center includes a large lake surrounded by more than 5 miles of trails along with an education and exhibit center. Bird blinds are located around the lake. The Capital Area Greenbelt follows the longest trail along the lake's west shore.

Connected to the greenbelt is the Walnut Street Bridge (also called People's Bridge), a restored iron trestle bridge that takes you from City Island to the riverfront walkway along Front Street in Harrisburg. Built in 1889, it was part of the city's street car system until 1950, when it was converted to automobile use. In 1972, Hurricane Agnes damaged the bridge beyond repair for vehicular use so it was converted to a pedestrian-only bridge. Icy floodwaters washed away the western span of the bridge in 1996; Rails-to-Trails Conservancy is assisting efforts to restore the structure. The eastern segment of the bridge has been reopened to pedestrians, and is well worth a visit. Its lack of completion is not an impediment to riding the greenbelt.

DIRECTIONS

To reach the Walnut Street Bridge on City Island, from Interstate 83, take the 2nd Street exit. Follow 2nd Street north to Market. Turn left. Follow Market across the bridge to City Island. You will see the City Island parking lot entrance on your right. The Walnut Street Bridge sits parallel and north of the Market Street bridge.

To reach Wildwood Lake Sanctuary, from Interstate 81, take Exit 66 for Front Street. Go north on Front Street to the first traffic light, and turn right onto Route 39 (Linglestown Road). Turn right at the first light onto Industrial Road. Go a little more than 1 mile, and turn left onto Wildwood Way. Follow the paved road until you come to the nature center parking lot.

The section beginning at City Island and running along Front Street is wheelchair-accessible.

Contact: Capital Area Greenbelt Association
P.O. Box 15405
Harrisburg, PA 17105
(717) 921-4733
www.caga.org

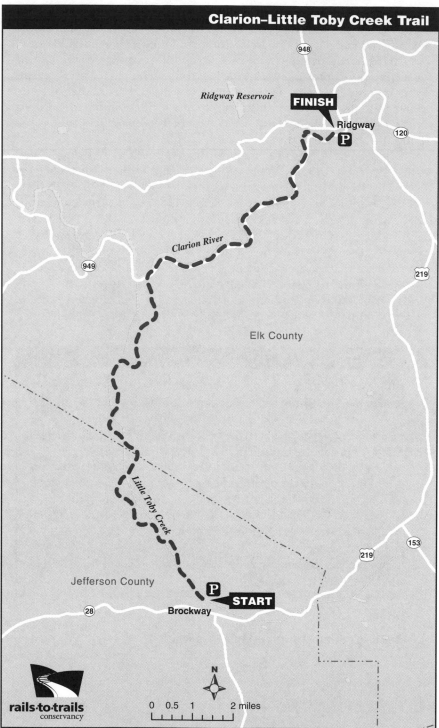

Clarion–Little Toby Creek Trail

948

Ridgway Reservoir

FINISH

Ridgway

P

120

949

Clarion River

219

Elk County

Little Toby Creek

153

219

Jefferson County

P

START

28

Brockway

N

rails·to·trails
conservancy

0   0.5   1   2 miles

Clarion–Little Toby Creek Trail

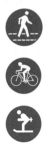

This picturesque trail meanders along the Wild and Scenic Clarion River and Little Toby Creek through Elk and Jefferson counties, between the charming small towns of Ridgway and Brockway. As you follow the trail, you are treated to spectacular mountain scenery and river vistas, possible wildlife sightings, and signs describing the area's history. You even cross Little Toby Creek on a swinging bridge.

The trail uses the former Clearfield to Ridgway Rail Company corridor, built in 1886 to transport lumber and coal from mills to markets but which also provided popular passenger service between Ridgway and Falls Creek. After the line ceased operation in the 1960s, Penn Central bought the corridor and ran trains there until 1968. The rail-trail opened in 1992.

Beginning in Brockway, this serene 18-mile trail, beginning in Brockway, travels through some true Pennsylvania wilderness and wildlands. The landscape is

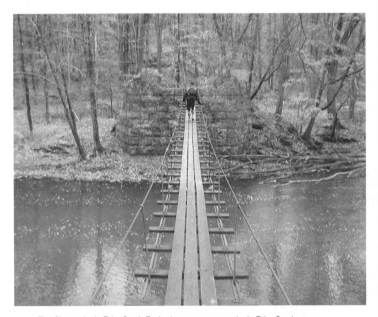

The Clarion–Little Toby Creek Trail takes users across Little Toby Creek on a swinging bridge.

Location
Elk and Jefferson counties

Endpoints
Ridgway to Brockway

Mileage
18

Roughness Index
1

Surface
Crushed stone and dirt

179

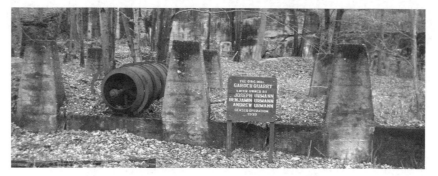

Spectacular mountain scenery, superb river vistas, wildlife, and signs describing the area's history can all be seen on the trail.

reminiscent of scenes from a James Fenimore Cooper novel. As the trail travels north, it follows Little Toby Creek through lush forested hills and breathtaking views of the wild creek. A little beyond the half-way point, you reach the confluence of the Little Toby Creek and the Clarion River. The trail follows the banks of the Clarion River until it reaches the endpoint in the town of Ridgway.

A 1.8-mile section of trail runs adjacent to a live railroad line, so be careful. The trail is located near the Allegheny National Forest. During hunting season, wear bright clothing—a fluorescent orange vest is best—and remain on the trail at all times. The tree cover provides shade in the summer months. Keep an eye out for deer, wild turkeys, herons, eagles and other wildlife.

DIRECTIONS

To reach the Brockway Trailhead, from Interstate 80 take Route 219 North into Brockway. Turn left onto Main Street, then right onto 7th Avenue. The trailhead is just past the community pool.

To reach the Ridgway Trailhead, from Interstate 80, take State Route 219 North to State Route 948 (Main Street) in Ridgway. Follow 948 through town and turn left on Water Street, just before Love's Canoe and Keystone Hardware. Continue one block to the trailhead.

Contact: TriCounty Rails to Trails Association
P.O. Box 115
Ridgway, PA 15853
www.pavisnet.com/tcrtt/

Clearfield to Grampian Trail

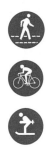

Take in scenic views of water, farmland and forests and a vibrant history of railroad commerce and Native American life. As you walk, bike or ski this easy and smooth trail from Clearfield to Grampian, you'll enjoy the glistening waters of Kratzer Run, Anderson Creek and the Susquehanna River. The former railroad line carried tons of coal and quarried stone along the East Coast, as well as clay, which was used to make bricks in the many brickyards along the trail.

Grampian, named by Scottish settlers after the Grampian Mountains of Scotland, was also home to Quakers in the early 1800s. Clearfield, settled in the late 1700s by Revolutionary War veterans with land grants, was named for the clearings made by grazing bison. The Native Americans called this major trading center along the Susquehanna River Chinklacamoose. The trail

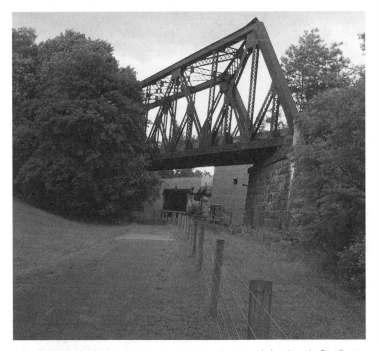

Location
Clearfield County

Endpoints
Clearfield to
Grampian

Mileage
10.5

**Roughness
Index**
2

Surface
Crushed limestone

Railroad bridges that once saw trains carrying coal, stone and clay along the East Coast are visible from the trail.

181

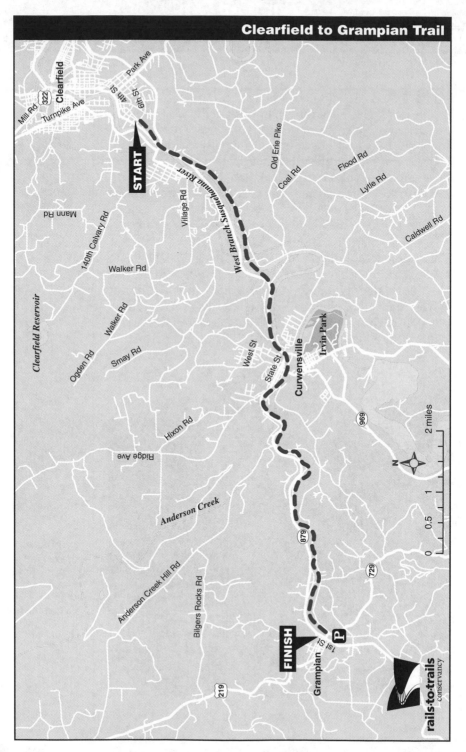

Clearfield to Grampian Trail

Clearfield
Mill Rd
322
Turnpike Ave
Park Ave
4th St
6th St
START
Old Erie Pike
Coal Rd
Flood Rd
Lytle Rd
Caldwell Rd
Mann Rd
Village Rd
West Branch Susquehanna River
140th Calvary Rd
Walker Rd
Ogden Rd
Walker Rd
Smay Rd
West St
State St
Curwensville
Irvin Park
Clearfield Reservoir
969
N
Hixon Rd
Ridge Ave
2 miles
1
0.5
0
Anderson Creek
879
729
Anderson Creek Hill Rd
Bilgers Rocks Rd
FINISH
1st St
P
Grampian
219
rails-to-trails
conservancy

was part of the Great Shamokin Path used by the Lenape and Mohican tribes.

This trail offers several opportunities for stops to enjoy the scenic beauty of the area with picnic tables available at around 2.5 miles, 4 miles, and 6.7 miles outside of Grampian. Several railroad bridges remind you of the railroad commerce that was important to the area when the railroad was built in the late 1860s and 1870s. The first two bridges you pass are located in the borough of Curwensville about 4 miles outside of Grampian.

DIRECTIONS

To reach the Clearfield Trailhead, take Interstate 80 to Exit 120 for Clearfield. Take Route 879 South about 2.5 miles, and turn right on the Spruce Street exit. Take the first left (Chester Street) and in another 200 yards, turn left. Parking is available at the trailhead.

The Grampian Trailhead is one block from the stoplight at the intersection of U.S. 219 and Routes 879 and 729. A large sign on Route 729 identifies the trailhead and public parking area.

Contact: Clearfield County Recreation and Tourism Authority
12 North Front Street
Clearfield, PA 16830
(814) 765-5734
www.clearfieldrailstotrails.com

Coal & Coke Trail

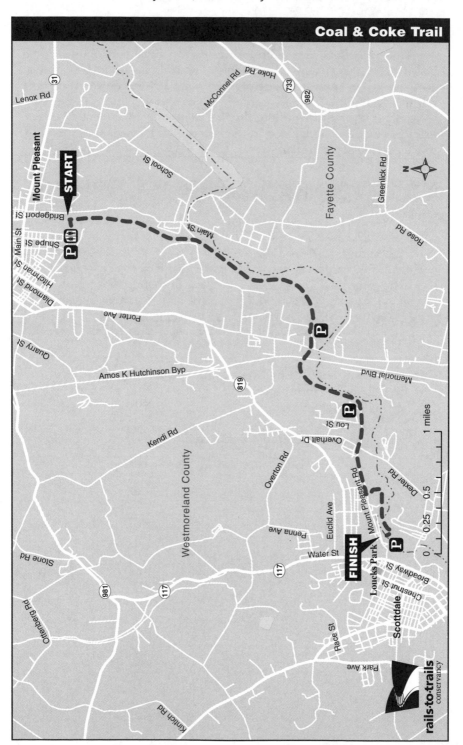

Coal & Coke Trail

The scenic Coal & Coke Trail connects the communities of Mount Pleasant and Scottdale in Westmoreland County and offers many glimpses of the picturesque nature and local communities of Westmoreland County. The 6-mile trail is built on the old Pennsylvania Railroad corridor, and sections parallel the active Southwest PA line toward Bridgeport. The old railroad corridor was used to transport coal and coke from the many coal mining companies in the county in the early 1900s. The trail finally opened in 2007 after eight years of planning and development.

Starting at Willows Park in Mount Pleasant, the trail runs through beautiful scenic wooded areas to the town of Bridgeport. Beyond Bridgeport, the trail quickly dips into woodlands again, and is lined with trees to Hammondville and Iron Bridge. From here the trail runs under US 119 and continues along the old Pennsylvania Railroad corridor to Mildred Street in North Scottdale.

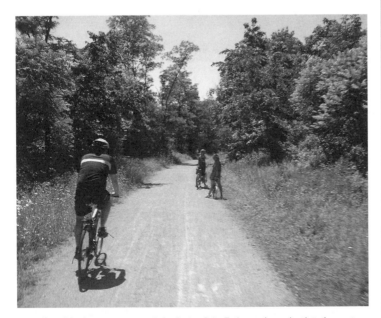

Named for the cargo it serviced, the Coal & Coke Trail is partly a rail-with-trail, occasionally running adjacent to an active rail line.

Location
Westmoreland County

Endpoints
Mount Pleasant to Scottdale

Mileage
6

Roughness Index
1

Surface
Crushed stone

185

You'll follow Mildred Street for five blocks to Kendi Park. You can stop here or take a sharp left after Kendi Park, and follow the Coal & Coke Trail for a quarter mile to its junction with the scenic milelong Jacob's Creek Multi-Use Trail that runs west toward Scottdale.

DIRECTIONS

To reach the Mount Pleasant Trailhead, from Interstate 76, take Exit 75 toward US 119 West and State Route 66 West toll road and merge with General Edward Martin Highway North. Take the US 119 South exit toward Connelsville. After 5 miles, take the exit toward Mount Pleasant/Ruffs Dale; after 1.4 miles turn left on State Route 31. Continue to South Silver Street and turn right. Then turn left on Spruce Street and take a right on Clay Avenue. The parking area will be on your left in Willows Park.

To reach the Scottdale Trailhead, from Interstate 76, take Exit 75 toward US 119 West and State Route 66 West toll road and merge with General Edward Martin Highway North. Take the US 119 South exit toward Connelsville. After 7.6 miles, take the Scottdale exit and merge unto State Route 819 and Porter Avenue. Turn left on 6th Street and take a right on Mount Pleasant Road North (Scottdale Road). There's plenty of parking at the park.

This trail is wheelchair-accessible.

Contact: Westmoreland County Bureau of Parks and Recreation
P.O. Box 360
Scottdale, PA 15683
www.co.westmoreland.pa.us/parks/cwp/view.
asp?A=3&Q=619363

Conewago Recreational Trail

T he Conewago Recreational Trail in northwestern Lancaster County parallels Conewago Creek over most of its length as it passes through farmland and forests. A unit of the Lancaster County Department of Parks and Recreation, the 5.1-mile trail occupies the former rail bed of the Cornwall-Lebanon Railroad from PA Route 230 near Elizabethtown to the Lebanon County line, where it joins the 14.5-mile Lebanon Valley Rail-Trail (see page 245).

Robert H. Coleman built the railroad in 1883 as a private venture, and the line operated for nearly a century. Trains transported iron ore to the Pennsylvania Railroad, which took it to the mill in Steelton. The railroad also ran passenger trains to and from Mt. Gretna, home of the Pennsylvania Chautauqua and the National Guard encampment for nearly a half century starting in 1885.

The well-graded crushed stone trail is suited for a variety of visitors, including pedestrians, cyclists and cross-country skiers. Numerous horse farms dot the trail, and equestrian use along the corridor is evident. There are only six road crossings; they are well-marked and usually involve low-volume rural roads.

From the trailhead on Pennsylvania Route 230, the trail heads northeast through the countryside. Over most of its length, the trail runs along the quiet, meandering Conewago Creek and through rich Lancaster County farmland. Most of the trail is shaded by trees that edge the fields and meadows.

The crossing of Mill Street, where the original railroad bridge has been removed, features sloped ramps down to the road level and back up to the trail. Use caution at this crossing since it's on a curve.

At the Lebanon County line where the Conewago Rail Trail joins the Lebanon Valley Rail-Trail, there is no trailhead access. Signs and a change of surface signify the transition from one trail to the other.

Location
Lancaster and
Lebanon counties

Endpoints
State Route 230
in Elizabethtown
to Lebanon
and Lancaster
County line

Mileage
5.1

**Roughness
Index**
2

Surface
Crushed stone

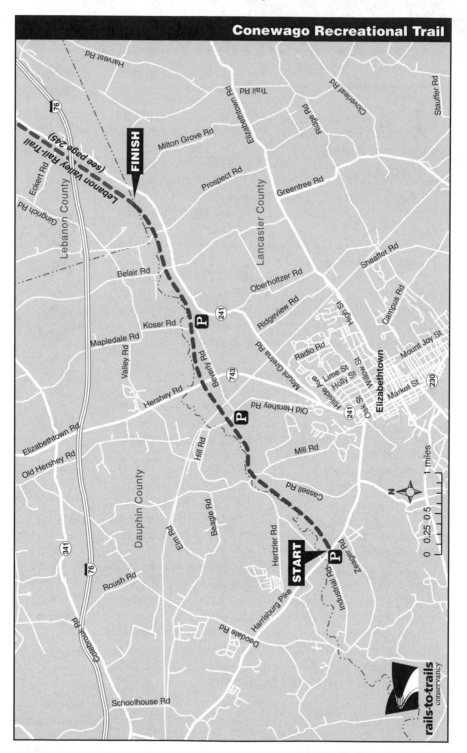

Conewago Recreational Trail

DIRECTIONS

To reach the State Route 230 Trailhead, from Elizabethtown, proceed northeast for approximately 2 miles on State Route 230 (North Market Street). The trailhead is on the right just before a bridge over Conewago Creek.

To other access points: State Route 241 (Mount Gretna Road) runs parallel to the trail over most of its length and provides access via rural side roads.

There are small parking areas (enough for a few cars) at most points where the trail intersects roads.

Contact: Lancaster County Parks and Recreation Department
1050 Rockford Road
Lancaster, PA 17602
(717) 295-8215
www.co.lancaster.pa.us/parks/site/default.asp

Corry Junction Greenway Trail

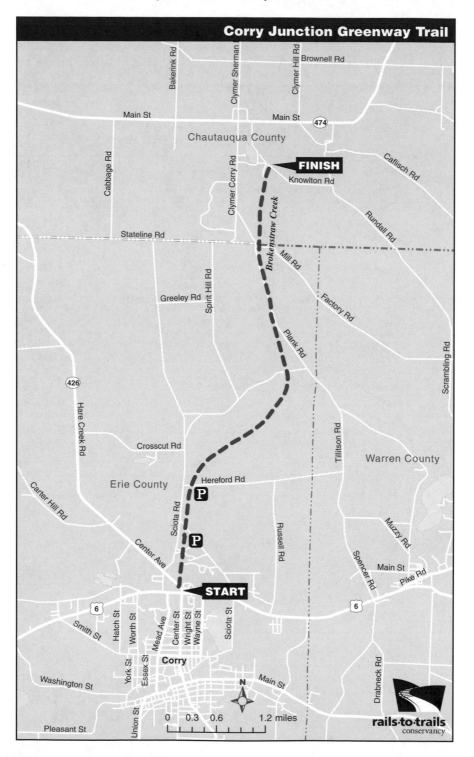

Chautauqua County

FINISH

Warren County

Erie County

Corry

0   0.3   0.6   1.2 miles

rails·to·trails
conservancy

Corry Junction Greenway Trail

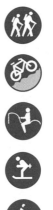

Corry Junction Greenway Trail
Trailhead Parking

Crossing the state line into New York near Erie, Pennsylvania, the 7.5-mile trail runs through the beautiful Brokenstraw Valley, passing small streams, a tamarack swamp, deciduous woods and wildflowers.

The construction of railroad tracks through the piney woods of northern Pennsylvania in the early 1800s heralded a new era. By 1861, the Atlantic & Great Western Railroad intersected the Sunbury & Erie Railroad at a spot called, appropriately enough, Junction. The land at Junction was owned by Hiram Cory, who sold a small piece of this 63-acre holding to the A&GW Railroad in October 1861. Railroad superintendent Hill was so pleased by Mr. Cory's fair price that he renamed Junction in his honor, although he misspelled it in the process. That was the beginning of the City of Corry.

In 1865 the Oil Creek Cross Cut Railroad from Oil City, Pennsylvania, across the state line to Mayville, New York, was completed The line operated under a number of different names until December 29, 1978, when the last train from Corry to Mayville ran on what was then called the Titus Secondary Tract. Included in

Location
Chautauqua, NY, and Erie, PA, counties

Endpoints
Corry, PA, to Clymer, NY

Mileage
7.5

Roughness Index
3

Surface
Dirt, crushed stone and grass

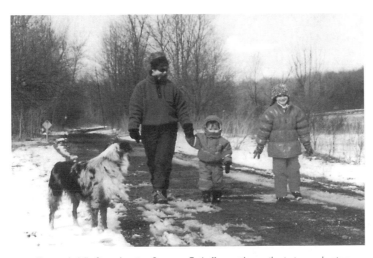

The rough, hilly Corry Junction Greenway Trail offers outdoor enthusiasts an adventure year-round.

191

Corry's rich railroad history is the invention and manufacturing of the Climax locomotive and rail cars that the logging industry used from 1888 until the 1920s. The Northwest Pennsylvania Trail Association purchased a portion of the rail corridor, from Corry to Clymer, in 2003.

The rough, hilly trail offers outdoor enthusiasts an adventure year-round. Several crossings do not meet the grade of the road or have inclines where cyclists may need to dismount. Transportation Enhancement funds (the largest source of federal funding for rail-trails) have been approved to make vast improvements to the trail surface, drainage and amenities such as trailheads and signage.

DIRECTIONS

To reach the Corry Trailhead in Pennsylvania, follow State Route 6 into downtown Corry. Turn north onto Sciota Street. The trail shares a dirt road access off to the right. There is limited public parking available in town.

To reach the southern trailhead in Pennsylvania—the only mid-trail trailhead that has parking—in Corry, turn north onto Route 426. Bear right onto Sciota Road and to Hereford Road. Turn right on Hereford Road. The trailhead is on the left.

Contact: Northwest Pennsylvania Trail Association
P.O. Box 9401
Erie, PA 16505
(814) 664-3884
www.nwpatrail.org

Cumberland County
Biker-Hiker Trail

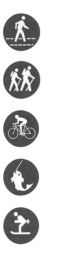

This gently winding trail in Pine Grove Furnace State Park passes along the shore of two lakes and through the woodlands of Michaux State Forest. Pine Grove Furnace began operating in 1764 to take advantage of the small but rich South Mountain iron ore deposits. The furnace closed in 1895 as new technology made the operation of small ironworks unprofitable. The 17,000-acre property of the South Mountain Ironworks was sold to the State of Pennsylvania in 1914 to become part of a new forest reserve system. Remnants of the days of iron production are evident in the park. The ironmaster's mansion, furnace ruins and other buildings provide a historical perspective.

The park's two lakes, 25-acre Fuller Lake and 1.7-acre Laurel Lake, are also remnants of the area's iron making heritage. Fuller Lake was an iron ore quarry that filled with groundwater when operations ceased. Laurel Lake provided water power to Laurel Forge,

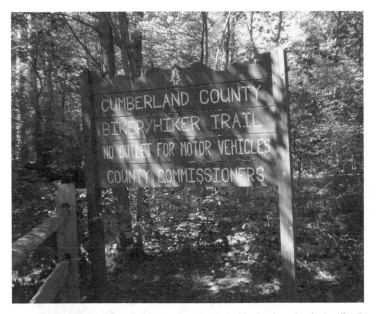

Pine Grove Furnace State Park houses historic industrial landmarks and is the "unofficial" halfway point of the Appalachian Trail.

Location
Cumberland County

Endpoints
Furnace Stack Day Use Area to Pine Grove Road and Old Railroad Bed Road in Pine Grove Furnace State Park

Mileage
2.2

Roughness Index
2

Surface
Asphalt, cinder and crushed stone

193

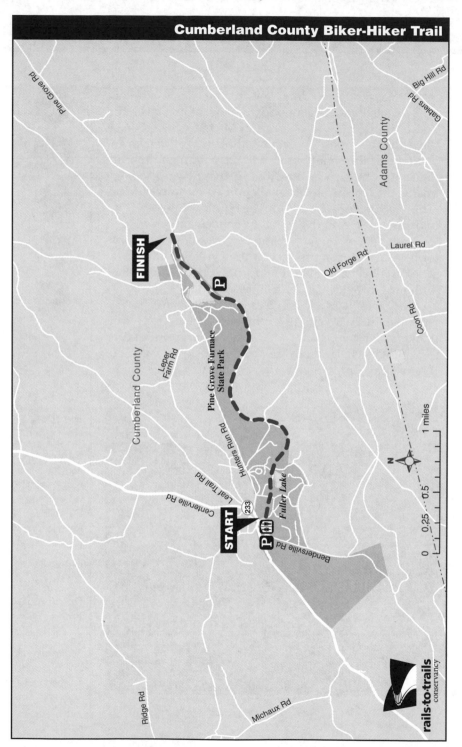

Cumberland County Biker-Hiker Trail

which produced wrought iron. Both lakes now provide opportunities for swimming and fishing. Boating is permitted on Laurel Lake, which has a launch area, mooring slips and boat rental. Only electric motors are permitted.

The trail follows the route of the South Mountain Railroad. Constructed in the late 1860s the railroad brought raw materials to the furnace at Pine Grove and delivered finished iron products to market.

Pine Grove Furnace State Park marks the "unofficial" halfway point along the Appalachian Trail. The historic ironmaster's mansion now serves as a hostel with dormitory style overnight accommodations and cooking and dining facilities.

The trail begins in the park at the Appalachian Trail parking lot near the Furnace Stack Day Use Area. A short paved section of trail leads from the parking area to the Fuller Lake area, which has a beach. Swimming is permitted from late May until mid-September. Beyond the lake, the trail crosses a small bridge and turns left. This section of the trail runs on a gravel service road bordered by a swamp on one side and Mountain Creek on the other. The service road is closed to all traffic except official park vehicles. At a gate, the trail opens onto Old Railroad Bed Road and shares the corridor with occasional automobiles.

After passing Laurel Lake, Old Railroad Bed Road intersects Pine Grove Road and the trail ends.

DIRECTIONS

To reach the Furnace Stack Day Use Area Trailhead—the best access point—from PA Route 233, take Pine Grove Road and turn onto Bendersville Road. Turn onto Quarry Road. Parking is available at the Appalachian Trail parking area.

Contact: Pine Grove Furnace State Park
1100 Pine Grove Road
Gardners, PA 17324
(717) 486-7174
www.visitPAparks.com

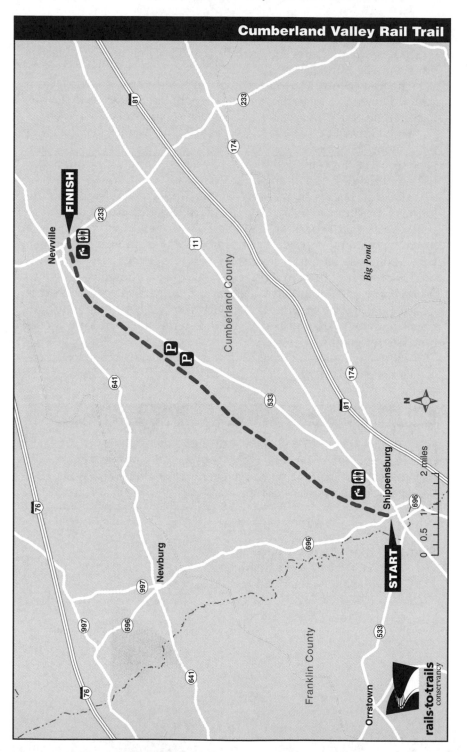

Cumberland Valley Rail Trail

Cumberland Valley Rail Trail

The Cumberland Valley Rail Trail runs down the middle of its namesake—the Cumberland Valley of Pennsylvania, between the South Mountain and Blue Mountain ridges on the eastern flank of the Appalachians. Stretching from New York State to Alabama, this lush agricultural valley formed a travel corridor for Native Americans, and for the Scotch-Irish immigrants who began settling here in the mid-1700s.

In the first half of the 19th-century railroad companies opened lines along the same route. Among them was the Cumberland Valley Railroad. Later owned by the Pennsylvania Railroad and then Conrail, which stopped using the corridor and donated it to The Cumberland Valley Rails-to-Trails Council for development of the breathtaking Cumberland Valley Rail Trail. It is interesting to note that the original engineers of the railroad did not want to use this selected route in the first place.

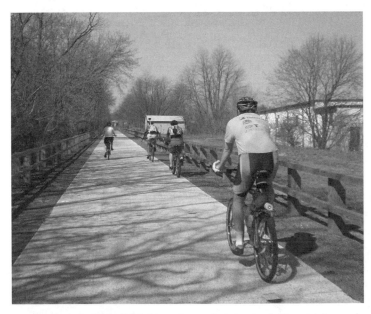

The Cumberland Valley Rail Trail has a firm, crushed-stone tread with good drainage and is often busy with cyclists on weekends.

Location
Cumberland County

Endpoints
Shippensburg Township Park in Shippensburg to McFarland Road in Newville

Mileage
10.9

Roughness Index
2

Surface
Crushed stone

Most of the well-designed trail runs fairly straight through open farmland, with a few dips into woodlands and some limestone out-croppings. It has good drainage and a firm, crushed-stone tread. You may see an occasional buggy from the surrounding Amish communi-ty on nearby country roads. Many Shippensburg University students and residents use the trail for jogging and walking. On the weekends it is active with cyclists.

At the Newville Trailhead, where PennDOT runs an instrument calibration facility and maintains a measured course on the trail, a half-mile section is paved with asphalt and cement. On the western end, the improved section of trail ends at Shippensburg Township Park. The right-of-way continues into the Shippensburg University campus, but it is unimproved and unsigned and includes a steep, dan-gerous road crossing. There are a few local eateries on the opposite side of the campus at the very end of the right-of-way.

The Cumberland Valley Rails-to-Trails Council hopes to install a crossing bridge in Shippensburg, which will provide a safe route along the entire right-of-way. Other plans are being considered to ex-tend the trail east from Newville.

Both the Newville and Shippensburg Township Park trailheads include restrooms and parking. The trailhead at the Shippensburg Township Park also accommodates horse trailers.

DIRECTIONS

To reach the Newville Trailhead, from the Harrisburg and Carlisle area, take PA Interstate 81 South. Take Exit 37 at Newville onto PA Route 233 North. Turn left onto PA Route 533 West. Follow 533 West through town, and turn left on Cemetery Road. Follow the road to where it ends at McFarland Street and the parking area.

To reach the Shippensburg Township Park trailhead, take Inter-state 81 to Exit 29. Turn right onto Walnut Bottom Road. Turn left onto King Street (US 11). Turn onto North Queen Street, then right onto Britton Road. The park is approximately a half mile ahead on the left.

All developed sections of the trail are wheelchair-accessible.

Contact: Cumberland Valley Rails-to-Trails Council
P.O. Box 531
Shippensburg, PA 17257
(717) 860-0444
www.cvrtc.org

D&H Rail Trail

The Delaware & Hudson (D&H) Gravity Railroad conducted a 3-mile test of the first steam locomotive in the U.S. in August 1829 from the towns of Honesdale to Seeleyville, Pennsylvania, and discovered that the train was too heavy for the track. By 1830, the D&H Railroad's 17 miles of track constituted the vast majority of total railroad tracks in the U.S. at the time—just 23 miles!

From these small beginnings, the D&H became a successful mining and railroad company, shipping anthracite coal and lumber from the Lackawanna Valley in northeastern Pennsylvania to the East Coast of the U.S. and to Canada. As the supply of coal and lumber were depleted from the area, the need for the railroad diminished, and the rail-trail came into being.

As the trail is comprised of cinder, original ballast, and hard-packed dirt, you need a hybrid or mountain bike to comfortably ride this intermittently rugged trail.

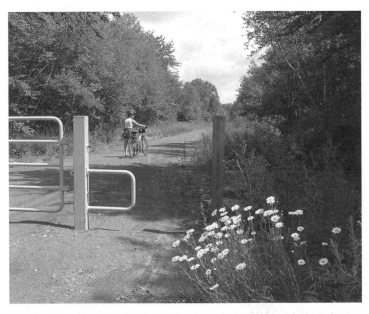

Because portions of the D&H Rail Trail have large chunks of ballast and steep inclines, cyclists may need to dismount.

Location
Lackawanna, Susquehanna and Wayne counties

Endpoints
Simpson to Stevens Point

Mileage
32

Roughness Index
3

Surface
Cinder, original ballast and packed dirt

199

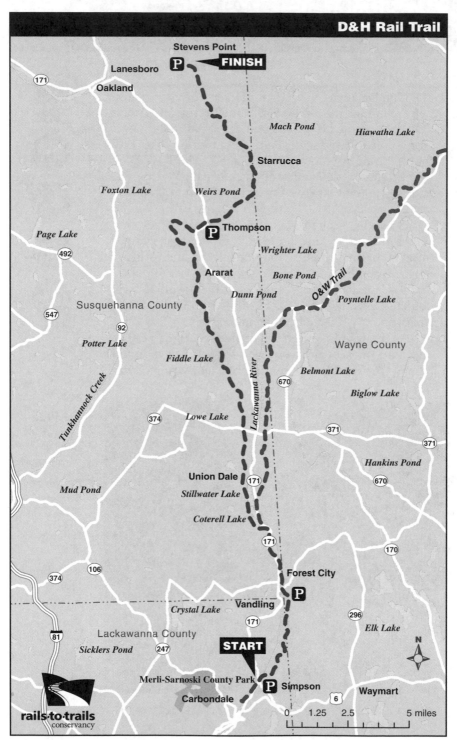

D&H Rail Trail

Stevens Point
Lanesboro
Oakland
171

FINISH

Mach Pond

Hiawatha Lake

Starrucca

Foxton Lake

Weirs Pond

Page Lake

492

Thompson

Wrighter Lake

Ararat

Bone Pond

Dunn Pond

O&W Trail

Poyntelle Lake

Susquehanna County

547

92

Potter Lake

Wayne County

Fiddle Lake

Lackawanna River

Belmont Lake

670

Biglow Lake

Tunkhannock Creek

374

Lowe Lake

371

371

Hankins Pond

670

Mud Pond

Union Dale
171

Stillwater Lake

Coterell Lake

171

170

374

106

Forest City

Crystal Lake
Vandling

171

296

Elk Lake

81

Lackawanna County

Sicklers Pond

247

START

Merli-Sarnoski County Park

Simpson

Waymart

Carbondale

6

0   1.25   2.5   5 miles

N

rails·to·trails
conservancy

There are a few short sections with large chunks of ballast and steep inclines where you may need to walk your bike.

The trail parallels the Lackawanna River for several miles, offering scenic vistas of the river and several small lakes. Some areas of the trail are tree-lined, but some are out in the open—wear sunscreen. You can also shoot off to the east on the O&W Trail where it meets the D&H south of Union Dale. From Simpson to Ararat, you'll be pedaling constantly because of the slight incline in the trail. But from Ararat to Stevens Point, you'll have a much easier ride as the trail's grade is at a slight decline.

In Thompson, take a break at the homemade ice cream shop right alongside the trail. As of July 2008, the completed portion of the trail ends at Burdock Hill in the town of Stevens Point. In the future, the trail is expected to continue past the New York State border.

DIRECTIONS

To access the trail from Simpson, take Interstate 81 to Exit 185, then Route 6 to Carbondale. After the town of Carbondale, turn left onto Route 171. Continue 1 mile, park on the right side of the viaduct, next to the military tank. Follow the O&W Trail for 2 miles, where it accesses the D&H to the west.

Contact: Rail-Trail Council of Northeast Pennsylvania
P.O. Box 123
Forest City, PA 18421
(570) 679-9300
www.nepa-rail-trails.org

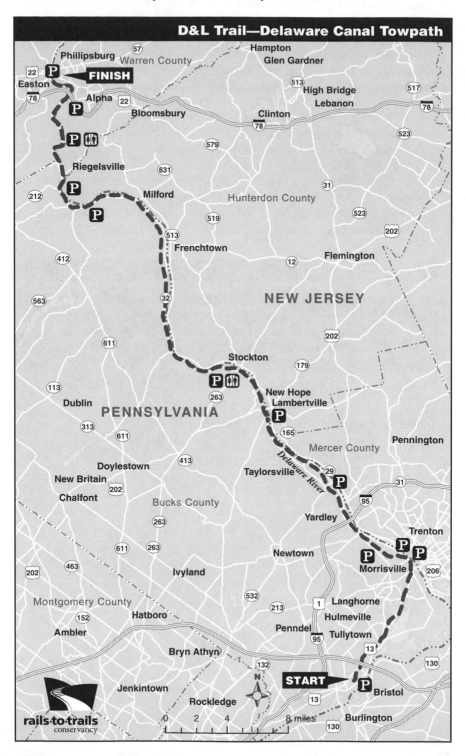

D&L Trail—Delaware Canal Towpath

D&L Trail–Delaware Canal Towpath

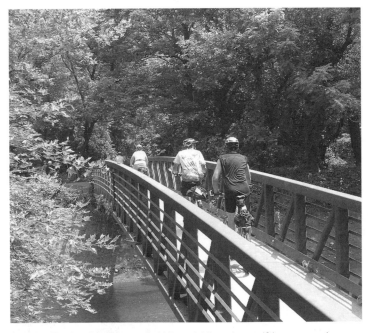

The Delaware Canal Towpath, which extends from Bristol to Easton, is the only continuously intact canal remaining from the historic canal-building era of the early and mid-1800s. Through its connection with the Lehigh Navigation Canal at Easton, the Delaware Canal helped to develop the anthracite coal industry in the Upper Lehigh Valley. In 1940 the canal system became a state park, and in 1988 Congress officially recognized the system's importance to the economic evolution of the U.S. by establishing the Delaware & Lehigh National Heritage Corridor.

Today the 60-mile Delaware Canal Towpath, once trod by teams of mules pulling cargo-laden boats, is one of four named trails that make up the 165-mile D&L Trail, the backbone of the National Heritage Corridor and the longest publicly owned trail remaining in the state. Other trails contained in the D&L are: the Lehigh

The 60 miles of the Delaware Canal Towpath follow a historic 19th-century canal.

Location
Bucks and
Northampton
counties

Endpoints
Bristol to Easton

Mileage
60

**Roughness
Index**
2

Surface
Crushed stone
and dirt

Gorge State Park Trail (see page 255), the Lehigh Canal: North (see page 249), and Lehigh Canal: South (see page 251).

Flood damage in 2004 and 2006 closed entire sections of the trail, but in July 2010, after millions of dollars in repair work, the entire trail has been reopened. Most of the repair work focused on the locks and canal itself. The trail surface remains bumpy with exposed tree roots; visitors should expect rough conditions.

A variety of looping routes can be followed using any of the five bridges that cross into New Jersey and connect to the Delaware and Raritan Canal State Park on the Jersey side of the river. Visitors can easily access both sides of the river exploring quaint towns, scenic river views and inland trails. Connecting bridges are in the Pennsylvania towns of Uhlerstown, Lumberville, Center Bridge, Washington Crossing and Morrisville.

DIRECTIONS

To reach the Washington Crossing Trailhead, from Interstate 95 to Exit 51 to New Hope. Stay left and merge onto Taylorsville Road. Travel 3 miles to Taylorsville, and turn right onto PA 532. Turn left on River Road (State Route 32). Park in the lot on the left.

Contact: Delaware Canal State Park
11 Lodi Hill Road
Upper Back Eddy, PA 18972
(610) 982-5560
www.dcnr.state.pa.us/stateparks/parks/delawarecanal.aspx

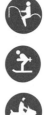

The Pennsylvania Railroad originally built the Chautauqua Line as part of a network of rail lines that linked Corry, Titusville, Oil City, Franklin and Meadville during the boom days of the oil industry in Northwest Pennsylvania. Spartansburg, Glynden and Centerville were important depots in the network. Heading south out of Spartansburg, the rail corridor parallels the East Branch of Oil Creek, hence the trail name.

After its establishment in 1988, the Clear Lake Authority purchased the 15.4-mile disused rail corridor to provide public access to Clear Lake in Spartansburg. Today a 7.5-mile section of the old railbed between Spartansburg and Centerville is used by hikers, hunters, snowmobilers, four-wheelers and horse-drawn Amish wagons. The flat East Branch is mostly ballast with some dirt. A small borough with a population of fewer than 300, Spartansburg is a commerce center to a sizable

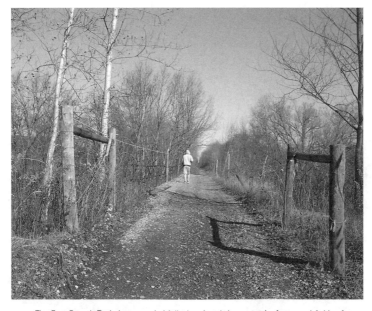

The East Branch Trail skirts wooded hillsides, Amish homesteads, farms and fields of brush to Clear Lake and nearby wetlands.

Location
Crawford County

Endpoints
Spartansburg to Centerville

Mileage
7.5

Roughness Index
1

Surface
Ballast

205

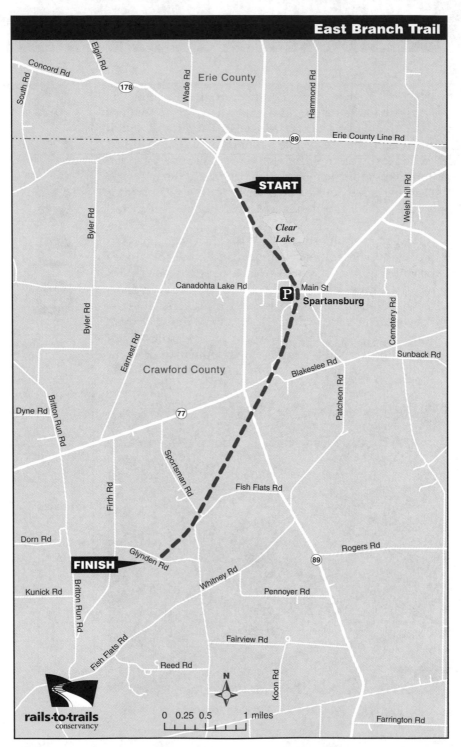

East Branch Trail

Erie County

Concord Rd
South Rd
Elgin Rd
178
Wade Rd
Hammond Rd
Erie County Line Rd
89
Welsh Hill Rd

◄ START

Clear Lake

Byler Rd

Canadohta Lake Rd
P Main St
Spartansburg
Cemetery Rd

Byler Rd

Earnest Rd

Crawford County

Blakeslee Rd
Sunback Rd
Patcheon Rd

Dyne Rd
Britton Run Rd
77

Sportsman Rd
Fish Flats Rd

Firth Rd

Dorn Rd
Rogers Rd
89
FINISH ◄
Glynden Rd

Kunick Rd
Britton Run Rd
Whitney Rd
Pennoyer Rd

Fish Flats Rd

Fairview Rd

Reed Rd
Koon Rd

N

rails·to·trails
conservancy

0   0.25 0.5   1 miles

Farrington Rd

Amish community. Horse-drawn buggies and wagons are a regular site in town and occasionally on the trail when it is used as an alternative transportation corridor, deemed safer than the main highways.

The trail skirts wooded hillsides, Amish homesteads, farms and fields of brush to Clear Lake and wetlands. Preservation of this corridor connects to Chautauqua County rail-trails in New York State and with Oil City, Pennsylvania, both areas that are filled with 19th- and 20th-century history and charm. Over the past decade Spartansburg has become a tourist destination for those in search of Amish furniture, antiques, country crafts and fresh maple syrup. Two bed–and-breakfasts are located in town, the Dutch Inn B&B and the Three Gable B&B, plus other accommodations to choose from. Clear Lake, which is actually a reservoir, offers canoeing and fishing. If you are interesting in fishing, consult local guides and resources.

The East Branch Trail is a key link in a system of trails that will eventually connect Lake Erie to the Chesapeake Bay via the Great Allegheny Passage (see page 221) and Erie to Harrisburg via the Mainline Canal Greenway. For more information about the East Branch Trail, please contact the Clear Lake Authority in Spartansburg.

DIRECTIONS

The trail can only be accessed in downtown Spartansburg at the parking area at the southern tip of Clear Lake, off Route 77 (Main Street). If you are heading east on Route 77, the parking area will be on your left.

Contact: Clear Lake Authority
P.O. Box 222
Spartansburg, PA 16434
(814) 664-7303 or (814) 654-2068
www.visitpa.com/visitpa/details.pa?id=222128+

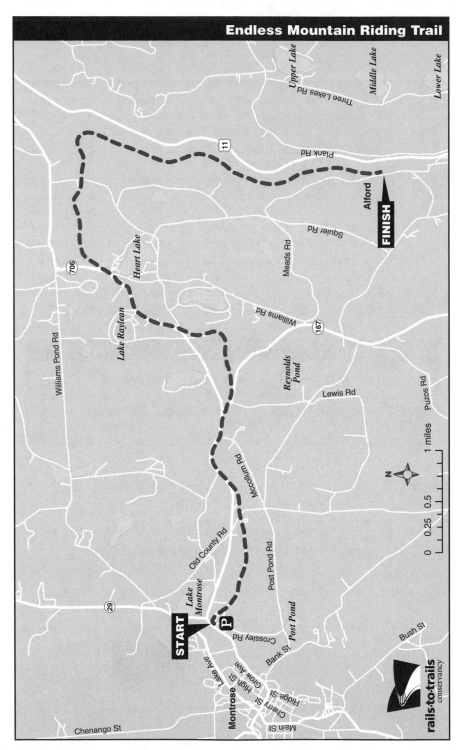

Endless Mountain Riding Trail

Endless Mountain Riding Trail

The local riding club enjoyed this former rail line, which was purchased in 1944 for a dollar from the Delaware, Lackawanna & Western Railroad, as a bridle trail for many years. It changed management over the years, and currently has no official manager. While this problem is expected to be remedied soon, the trail currently reflects the lack of oversight; there are no signs to the trail or through unclear road crossings. However, this pretty trail is fun to explore if you are game, whether by mountain bike, on horseback or on foot.

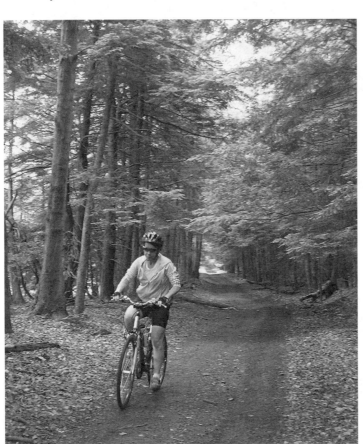

Who knew endless fun could cost only $1—the amount paid to buy the former rail line in 1944 for trail use.

Location
Susquehanna County

Endpoints
Behind the Pump & Pantry Convenience Store on State Route 706 in Montrose and the active rail line near Alford

Mileage
14

Roughness Index
3

Surface
Ballast and dirt

Starting in Montrose, the first 4 miles are rough-and-tumble, with sharp turns, exposed tree roots, large rocks, mud puddles, low-hanging branches and the occasional ATV user coming round the bend. The trail is narrow along much of this segment—shrinking to a two-foot path in places—which adds to the challenge, but also the fun.

At the second road crossing (State Highway 167) the trail continuation is obscured; look for it between two houses across the road, a little to the right. At the next road crossing, the trail continuation again is not obvious, but you should be able to find it if you cross the road and go to the left slightly, and down a gravel road about 500 yards.

For the next 6 miles the trail flanked by tall trees widens to two tracks, making more room for passing equestrians, cyclists or ATVs. A meager waterfall spills over the high bank on the right side at mile 8, but most of the water has been diverted to another course since the last flood. For the last 4 miles the trail courses gradually toward lower ground, and eventually ends at a working railroad nearly a mile from Alford. Since you cannot cross the railroad, you will need to head back up the trail to the starting point.

DIRECTIONS

To reach the access point in Montrose from Interstate 81, take Exit 223 west onto US 11 toward New Milford. Follow it about 2 miles through New Milford until State Route 706 West splits off to the right (north) and heads toward Montrose. Follow State Route 706 to the east side of town. Just past the golf course, turn left into the Pump & Pantry Convenience Store parking lot. The unmarked trailhead is behind the store on the left. The store staff are helpful if you have questions.

Contact: Rail-Trail Council of Northeast PA
P.O. Box 123
Forest City, PA 18421
(570) 679-9300

Ernst Bike Trail

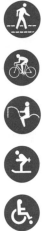

Along its 5-mile path, this paved rail-trail crosses through a rich array of natural habitats, from creek bottomlands to meadow, marsh and forest. The trail is named for Calvin Ernst, who owned the Meadville-Linesville Railroad corridor and donated it to French Creek Recreational Trails in 1996 for trail development.

Constructed from 1880 to 1892, the rail line connected Meadville to the Pennsylvania Railroad at Linesville. Business languished, and Bessemer & Lake Erie Railroad Company leased the corridor in 1891, using it to carry passengers to Exposition Park. Automobiles drove the rail route out of business in 1934; the line fell into disuse.

Traversing terrain with imprints of ice age glaciations, the trail follows the lush bottomlands of French Creek Valley. With 66 species of fish and 27 species of mollusks, the creek is the state's most biologically

Location
Crawford County

Endpoints
Meadville to
Watson Run

Mileage
5

Roughness Index
1

Surface
Asphalt

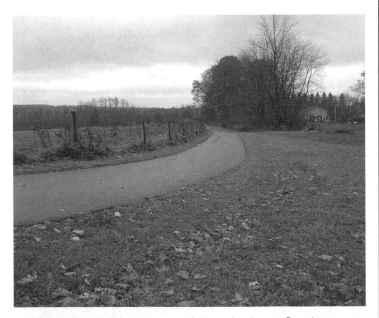

After the first mile, trail users are surrounded by rural northwestern Pennsylvania countryside.

211

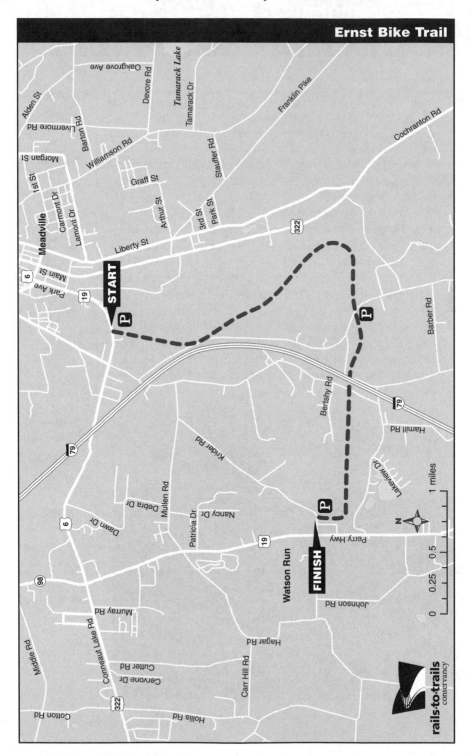

Ernst Bike Trail

diverse body of water. From the creek the trail passes through varied environments of meadow and marsh, hardwood stands and hemlock thickets.

Starting out at the Route 322 Trailhead in the busy commercial district of Meadville, the trail travels south following the peaceful banks of French Creek. You pass farmland and wooded areas in the first mile. Once you reach the Mercer Pike Trailhead, which is about halfway, you will have forgotten the hustle and bustle of Route 322 and be completely surrounded by rural northwestern Pennsylvania countryside. The trail gently turns west and crosses underneath Interstate 79. The trail continues for another mile before ending at the trailhead near Route 19.

There are plans to extend this trail to 11 miles, running to Conneaut Lake and Bicentennial Park. The new segment will run along Conneaut Marsh, a stopping point for many species of migrating waterfowl and home to bald eagles.

DIRECTIONS

To reach the Route 322 Trailhead, from Interstate 79, take Exit 147 (Routes 322 and 6) and head west for about 0.75 mile. The trailhead will be marked on your right. Pay close attention to the signs in this busy commercial area; the trailhead sign can be difficult to spot among the big box store signs.

To reach the Mercer Pike Trailhead, from the intersection of Route 322 and Mercer Pike, take Mercer Pike south. To stay on the pike, turn left prior to crossing Interstate 79, then follow Mercer Pike for 2 miles until it intersects with the bike trail. Parking is on the northwest side of the trail.

To reach the Route 19 Trailhead, from Interstate 79, take Exit 147 (Routes 322 and 6) and head east for about a mile. Take a left onto Route 19 and follow it south for close to 1.75 miles. The trailhead will be marked on the left.

This trail is wheelchair-accessible.

Contact: French Creek Recreational Trails, Inc.
P.O. Box 592
Meadville, PA 16335
(814) 724-6073
www.ernsttrail.org

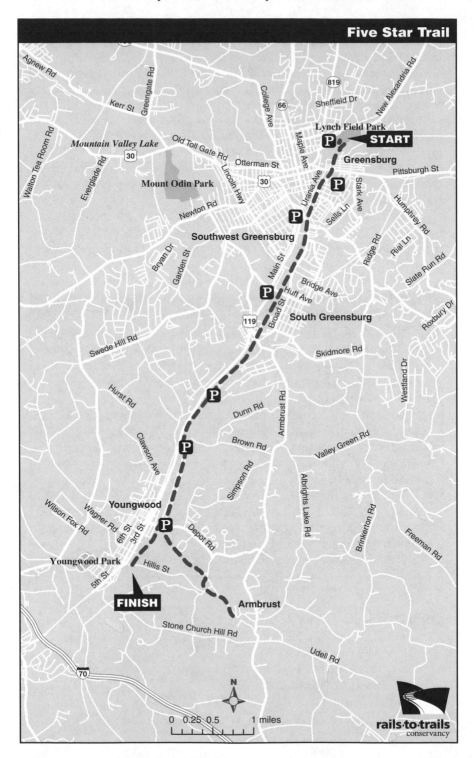

Five Star Trail

Agnew Rd

Kerr St

Greengate Rd

Walton Tea Room Rd

Mountain Valley Lake

30

Everglade Rd

Old Toll Gate Rd

Lincoln Hwy

College Ave

66

819

Sheffield Dr

New Alexandria Rd

Lynch Field Park

P

START

Greensburg

Pittsburgh St

Otterman St

30

Maple Ave

Urania Ave

P

Stark Ave

Humphrey Rd

Mount Odin Park

Newton Rd

Sells Ln

Ridge Rd

Rial Ln

Slate Run Rd

P

Southwest Greensburg

Bryan Dr

Garden St

Main St

Bridge Ave

Roxbury Dr

P

Huff Ave

Broad St

119

South Greensburg

Skidmore Rd

Westland Dr

Swede Hill Rd

P

Armbrust Rd

Hurst Rd

Dunn Rd

Valley Green Rd

P

Brown Rd

Clawson Ave

Simpson Rd

Albrights Lake Rd

Brinkerton Rd

Freeman Rd

Wilson Fox Rd

Wagner Rd

Youngwood

P

6th St

3rd St

Depot Rd

Youngwood Park

5th St

Hillis St

FINISH

Armbrust

Stone Church Hill Rd

Udell Rd

70

N

0   0.25 0.5   1 miles

rails·to·trails
conservancy

Five Star Trail

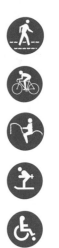

Trail users on this inviting corridor follow the path of an old Southern Pennsylvania Railroad line, in some places traveling alongside unused tracks. Riding the trail makes for a nice afternoon outing, combining pleasant scenery and historical attractions.

The trail runs nearly 8 miles through Westmoreland Country, extending south from Greensburg to Youngwood and then eastward to Armbrust. The Westmoreland County Industrial Development Corp. purchased the trail corridor from Conrail in 1995. The Westmoreland County Parks and Recreation Department is a partner in this project along with the municipalities of Greensburg, South Greensburg, Southwest Greensburg, Youngwood and Hempfield. The trail's name honors these fives municipalities. PA Cleanways keeps the trail clean.

Park at Lynch Field, a sports complex in Greensburg. The trail branches off to the east. Before embarking on

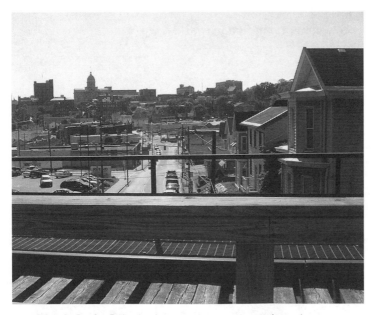

Riding the Five Star Trail makes for a nice afternoon outing, combining pleasant scenery and historical attractions.

Location
Westmoreland County

Endpoints
Greensburg to Armbrust

Mileage
7.7

Roughness Index
1

Surface
Crushed stone

215

this last 2-mile section, you may wish to stop in the Youngblood Trail Station, a museum focused on local railroad history. You will cross the campus of Westmoreland County Community College, along with a little park that features a pool, a playground and a few war relics, including an Apache helicopter.

At the south end, the trail splits at Depot Street. The short 1.5-mile stretch is paved and makes for a scenic walk or ride. Along the main trail, you'll see old rail cars and a converted caboose, once used as a restaurant.

DIRECTIONS

Access points are located off Route 119 beginning in Greensburg at Lynch Field, and continuing south to Huff Avenue, Willow Crossing Road, Trolley Line Avenue (Buncher Commerce Park), and finally Depot Street in Youngwood. At the Westmoreland County Community College, the trailhead is located on College Avenue across from the baseball field.

Contact: Westmoreland County Parks and Recreation
194 Donohoe Road
Greensburg, PA 15601
(724) 830-3950
www.co.westmoreland.pa.us/parks/cwp/view.
asp?a=3&q=619440

Ghost Town Trail

Despite its eerie name, there's nothing scary about the Ghost Town Trail. The trail is named for the numerous towns that were served by the Ebensburg & Backlick Railroad, as well as the Cambria & Indiana Railroad. It winds through scenic Blacklick Creek watershed from Ebensburg to Grafton, passing historical artifacts and offering opportunities to see a variety of wildlife. The trail, originally established in 1991, is a designated National Recreation Trail.

If you hit the trail early enough, you're likely to encounter deer and more than a few chipmunks. Once the sun gets high, watch out for the occasional snake sunning itself on the warm pathway.

A few interpretive signs along sections of the trail provide information about the mining towns, as well as some of the historical features. Mining slag and old railroad ties can be found at numerous points along the trail. Just west of Vintondale, you come to Eliza Furnace,

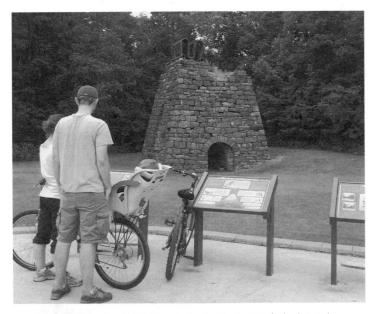

Interpretive signs along the trail describe local mining towns and other historical landmarks.

Location
Cambria and Indiana counties

Endpoints
Ebensburg to Grafton

Mileage
36

Roughness Index
1

Surface
Crushed stone and asphalt

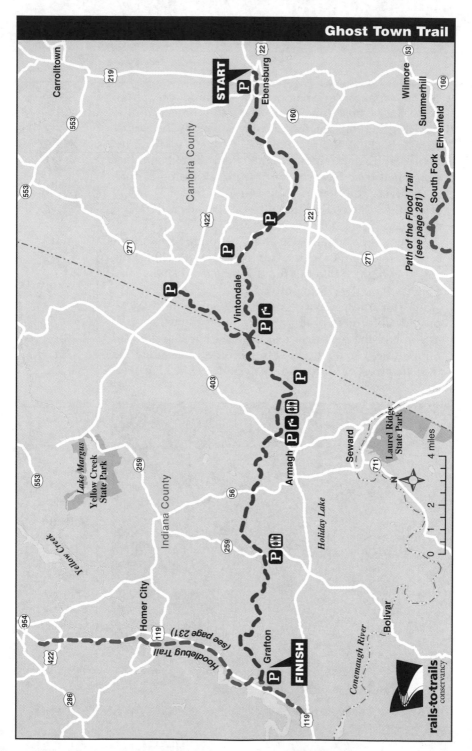

on the National Register of Historic Places and one of Pennsylvania's best preserved iron blast furnaces. East of Saylor Park, the trail passes a salvage yard of discarded rail cars. They make for a pleasant surprise, as the rusted hulks seem to bloom among the trees. In 2009 two beautiful bridges were installed to cross the Blacklick Creek west of Dilltown, one of the most popular trailheads along the route.

Some portions run though game lands—wear orange during hunting season. Bring your camera along to capture the natural beauty and historical features that you'll encounter during your visit. At the west end of the trail in Saylor Park, you may follow signs to connect to the Hoodlebug Trail (see page 231).

DIRECTIONS

To reach the Ebensburg Trailhead, from Altoona, take Route 22 west to Ebensburg, and turn right onto South Center Street. The street snakes left and then right. Before it veers right, you will see the trailhead and parking straight ahead.

To reach the Grafton Trailhead, from Altoona, take Route 22 west to Highway 119. Head north on 119. Proceed approximately 2 miles and turn right onto Main Street. Turn left onto Burrell Street. Parking is available across from the ball fields on Burrell Street, and the trailhead is visible at the end of the street.

This trail is wheelchair-accessible.

Contact: Indiana County Parks & Trails
1128 Blue Spruce Road
Indiana, PA 15701
(724) 463-8636
www.indianacountyparks.org/trails/gtt/gtt.html

Cambria County Conservation & Recreation Authority
401 Candlelight Drive, Suite 234
Ebensburg, PA 15931
(814) 472-2110
www.co.cambria.pa.us/Pages/Home.aspx

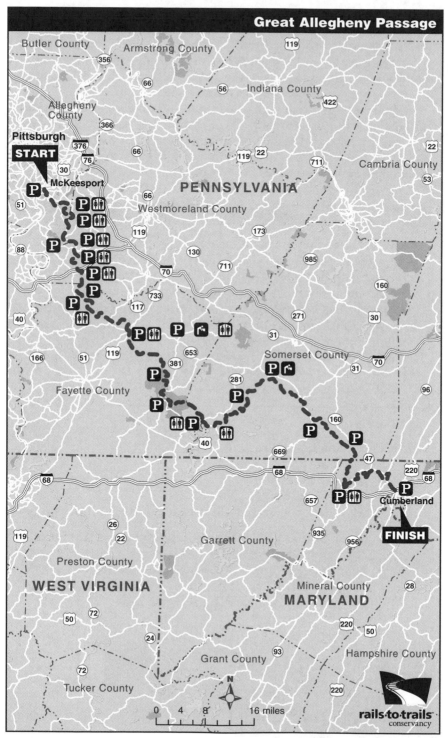

Great Allegheny Passage

N ow the longest rail-trail east of the Mississippi River, the 150-mile Great Allegheny Passage spans two states in its course along majestic rivers and across mountain passes. Running from Pittsburgh, Pennsylvania, to Cumberland, Maryland, the Great Allegheny Passage traces the paths of railroads that helped build America.

In 2010 the trail finalized agreements for the last mile of trail to be developed leading into Pittsburgh. After connecting with the Southside Trail, the trail heads south through McKeesport along the banks of the Youghiogheny River, following the route of the Pittsburgh, McKeesport and Youghiogheny Railroad. Built in 1883, the railroad carried coal and coke from the rich Connellsville District to the Pittsburgh steel mills. Nicknamed the P-Mickey for its initials, P. McK. & Y., it merged with the Pittsburgh and Lake Erie Railroad. The freight and coal traffic that sustained the branch dried up by the mid-1980s, and the line fell into disuse in 1990.

As you move upstream along the riverside trail, you pass lush green hillsides and once booming industrial towns. The first 40 miles of trail go through the Pennsylvania towns of Boston, West Newton and Dawson.

Location
Allegheny, Fayette, Somerset, Washington and Westmoreland counties

Endpoints
Pittsburgh, Pennsylvania, to Cumberland, Maryland

Mileage
135

Roughness Index
1

Surface
Crushed stone

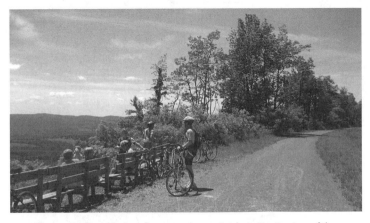

When on the Great Allegheny Passage, make sure to take in stunning views of the surrounding hills and agricultural valleys.

Trailside bed-and-breakasts, bike shops and cafes line the trail in these towns, making them great resting places.

At mile 43 the trail reaches the historic boomtown of Connellsville. This self-proclaimed "trail town" offers wonderful parks, restaurants and cafes. The industrial revolution is still alive in this southwestern Pennsylvania town.

For the next 17 miles, the trail follows the Youghiogheny River through remote Pennsylvania hill country. Take refuge under the dense canopy of the hardwood forest on the river's edge. Before reaching quaint Ohiopyle, you enter the state park with the same name and cross two impressive trestles. The town is a home base for adventure seekers. Not only is the trail a central attraction, but the Youghiogheny River is wild and untamed here and a popular whitewater rafting destination. Not even George Washington was able to navigate its rapids here; he was forced to turn around while trying to capture Fort Duquesne in 1754.

The trail continues south along the river for the next 11 miles to Confluence. Aptly named, the town is built where the Youghiogheny River, Casselman River and Laurel Hill Creek come together. It has plenty of great places to eat or catch a good night's rest.

South of Confluence the trail leaves the Youghiogheny and heads northeast for 31 miles, following the Casselman River to Meyersdale. You pass through the 849-foot-long Pinkerton tunnel in this stretch before getting to town. A pleasant old trailside train depot in Meyersdale provides good local information.

Be prepared to go uphill from here, as the trail heads southeast toward the Eastern Continental Divide. Here the trail follows the

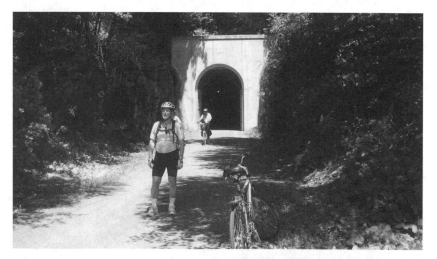

Several tunnels can be found on the trail, most notably the Pinkerton and Big Savage tunnels.

route of the old Western Maryland Railroad, which began operation between Cumberland, Maryland, and Connellsville, Pennsylvania, in 1912. Sold to a competitor in 1931, the railroad was operational for many more years before falling into disuse.

You cross the Eastern Continental Divide just before reaching the Maryland state line. From this elevation, more than 3,000 feet, it's all downhill to Cumberland. Pass through the half-mile-long Big Savage Tunnel just beyond the divide and take in stunning views of the surrounding hills and agricultural valleys as you pass the Mason-Dixon Line into Maryland, just beyond the tunnel. Frostburg is the first town you reach, about 5 miles into Maryland.

The trail leaves Frostburg and continues another 16 miles through rolling Maryland countryside to Cumberland. For much of this section, the trail parallels an active railroad line that is used for tourism. Cumberland, the terminus of the Great Allegheny Passage, does not disappoint. A pedestrian mall downtown has many restaurants and shops. In Cumberland, the trail connects to the Chesapeake and Ohio Canal National Historic Park towpath, which takes you another 184 miles to Washington, D.C., without ever leaving a trail.

DIRECTIONS

To reach the McKeesport Trailhead outside of Pittsburgh, Pennsylvania, from Pittsburgh, take Route 837 south out of the city and follow signs to McKeesport. Cross the McKeesport Duquesne Bridge, and pick up Route 837 (Lysle Boulevard) toward McKeesport. Follow 837 into town and veer onto the Water Street ramp on your right. Take a left onto Water Street. Parking for the trail is located in the park.

To reach the Cumberland Trailhead in Maryland, traveling west on Interstate 68 into Cumberland, take Exit 43B. Upon exiting, take a left onto West Harrison Street and then a right onto South Mechanic Street. The old Western Maryland train depot on your left has public parking for the trail.

Consulting the Allegheny Trail Alliance web page is the best bet for finding the many other access points on this long trail.

Contact: Allegheny Trail Alliance
P.O. Box 501
Latrobe, PA 15650
(888) 282-2453
www.atatrail.org

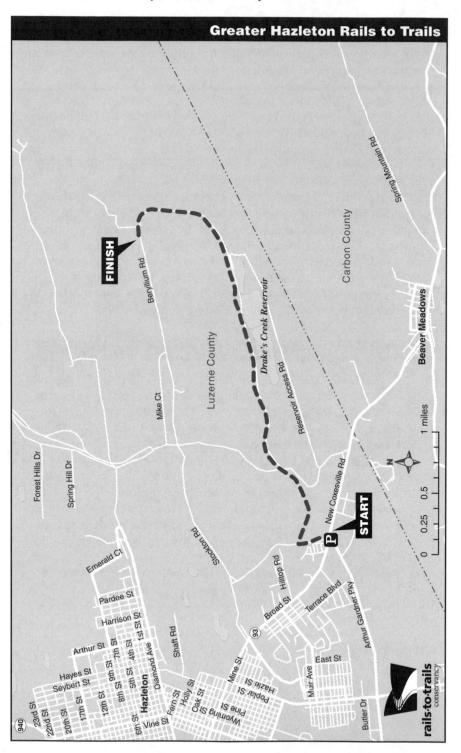

Greater Hazleton Rails to Trails

Greater Hazleton Rails to Trails

Like so many trails in this area, this trail occupies the former corridor of a railroad line that supported the local coal mining industry. After a half century of disuse, the local community has turned the corridor into a source of community pride. Today the trail runs 4 miles, but eventually it will be 16.4 miles and serve as a critical connection in the Delaware Lehigh National Heritage Corridor Trail system.

This trail is well maintained and flat throughout, with a crushed limestone surface perfect for walking and biking. It has nice amenities including good signs, mile markers, and parking facilities with trail maps. Keep in mind, however, that the trail dead-ends onto Beryllium Road, a decaying old paved road that you can't find on any map. So, although the route is 4 miles, it's best to consider it an 8-mile ride out and back until the planned trail extensions are complete.

The trail is well maintained, with frequent residential access points during the first mile. You'll find locals strolling, walking their dogs or getting in a quick jog. This trail is a popular place for geocaching, a game of hiding and seeking treasures with your GPS unit—particularly in the months when foliage is light, given that the trail is predominately tree-lined, with most sections covered in tree canopy. If you are looking to get a little more exercise, check out the five permanent exercise stations along the first mile. There is only one major road crossing before the 1-mile mark, and it is well signed. At about mile 2.5, the trail briefly loses its tree cover and picks up water views as it runs alongside Drake's Creek Reservoir. At the end of the reservoir, enjoy a scenic overlook and picnic table. From here the trail winds back into the woods and is less populated than the first half. You'll see an occasional path leading into a few neighboring communities as the trail winds down and dead-ends on Beryllium Road.

Location
Luzerne County

Endpoints
Intersection of State Routes 93 and 424 to Beryllium Road

Mileage
4

Roughness Index
1

Surface
Crushed stone

DIRECTIONS

From Interstate 81 on the south side of Hazleton, take Exit 141 turning right onto 4242 Arthur Gardner Parkway. Travel east approximately 4 miles until it dead-ends at State Road 93. Turn left at the 93 intersection. The trail entrance and parking lots are immediately on your right and well marked by a large sign.

This entire trail is wheelchair-accessible.

Contact: Greater Hazleton Civic Partnership
Citiscape
20 West Broad Street
Hazleton, PA 18201
(570) 455-1509
www.civicpartnership.com/railstotrails.html

Greene River Trail

About 60 miles south of Pittsburgh, the beautiful Greene River Trail parallels the Monongahela River as it winds through the coal mining region of Greene County. Conrail originally used the rail corridor until the Greene County Department of Recreation transformed the corridor into a striking nature trail, opened in 2001.

Driving through the river valley to the trail, you can glimpse several large coal mining operations just over the east ridge of the river. Remnants of older mine operations that processed and loaded coal onto railroad cars and river barges can still be seen along the trail; it's easy to imagine the days of old when barges ran up and down the Monongahela River to transport coal to the Ohio and Allegheny rivers in Pittsburgh.

The 5.2-mile trail starts in Millsboro at the Green Cove Yacht Club Trailhead. Once on the trail you follow Ten Mile Creek for less than a mile to where it flows into the Monongahela River. From there, the trail runs south along the river through a stretch of peaceful, scenic woodlands. The smooth trail surface is well maintained, and the trail is enclosed by rustic wood fencing

Location
Greene County

Endpoints
Millsboro to Crucible

Mileage
5.2

Roughness Index
1

Surface
Crushed stone

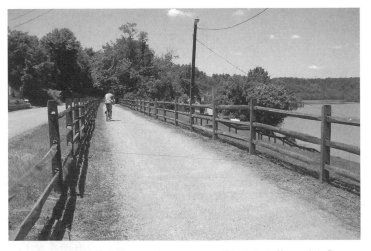

The Greene River Trail offers many sweeping views of the majestic Monongahela River and glimpses of the beautiful nature of Greene County.

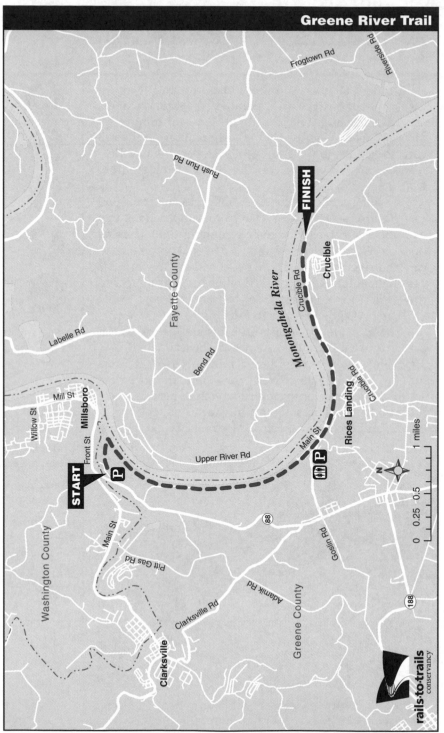

along much of the route. You'll encounter many sweeping views of the majestic Monongahela River and glimpses of the beautiful nature and peaceful surroundings of Greene County.

At about mile 3, you enter the town of Rices Landing. As you enter the township, you pass W. A. Young & Sons Foundry and Machine Shop, a restored, working 19th-century machine shop open to the public during the summer. Rices Landing, directly on the riverbank, offers a few local amenities to take a break for refreshments or a small bite to eat. You can also to begin your ride from the Rices Landing Trailhead.

After Rices Landing, the trail continues to wind along the Monongahela River for another 2 miles until you reach the endpoint along Crucible Road in Crucible. The trail ends abruptly in Crucible but will eventually extend another 9 miles to Nemacolin.

DIRECTIONS

To reach the Millsboro Trailhead, from State Route 40 take State Route 88 south along the Monongahela River. South of East Millsboro, Route 88 crosses Ten Mile Creek on an Iron Bridge. Cross the bridge and turn left into Greene Cove Marina at the end of the bridge. Follow the trail sign to the parking lot at the northern end.

To reach the Rices Landing Trailhead, from Route 40 take Route 88 south along the Monongahela River. Take Route 88 to the town of Dry Tavern. Turn east on State Route 1008. Continue to Rices Landing and look for the signs for the Greene River Trail. There are several parking areas and public restroom facilities at the Rices Landing Trailhead.

This trail is wheelchair-accessible.

Contact: Greene County Department of Recreation
107 Fairgrounds Road
Waynesburg, PA 15370
(724) 852-5323
www.co.greene.pa.us/secured/gc2/depts/rec/index.htm

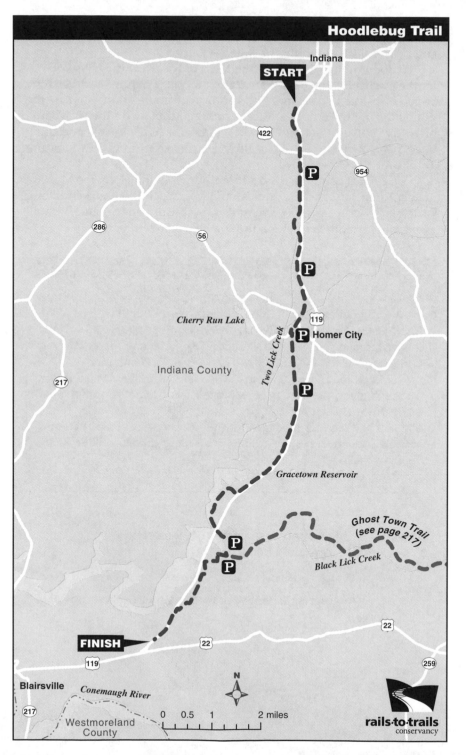

Hoodlebug Trail

Hoodlebug Trail

Any trail with a name like "Hoodlebug" deserves a visit. The 10-mile trail follows the path of the 1856-era Indiana Branch of the Pennsylvania Railroad, which ran from Blairsville north to the town of Indiana. "Hoodlebug" was the local nickname for the self-propelled passenger coach that traveled on the line until 1940.

The trail corridor has played an important role in the region for many years: as part of an extensive network of Native American trails, as a Pennsylvania Railroad branch line, and now as a pedestrian and bicycle trail used for both recreation and commuting by local residents and visitors to the area.

Today the trail, surfaced in part with highway millings provided by a partnership between Indiana County Parks and District 10 of the Pennsylvania Department of Transportation, also provides transportation options

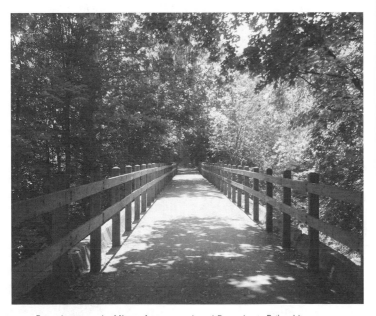

Formerly a network of Native American trails and Pennsylvania Railroad line, the Hoodlebug Trail continues to play an important role in the region.

Location
Indiana County

Endpoints
Indiana to Black Lick

Mileage
10

Roughness Index
2

Surface
Gravel

for commuters and university students and recreational opportunities along a historic corridor.

A dense forest of mixed deciduous and conifer trees lines most of the trail and provids a fine canopy on hot summer days. In contrast, the southern half of the trail passes rural and suburban homes along the State Route 119 corridor and follows a sound barrier wall. South of Homer City, as the trail crosses into Cambria County for its last mile, it parallels Two Lick Creek and becomes more rural.

Lengthened by 3 miles in 2005 as part of the Route 119 highway improvement project, in 2010 the Hoodlebug Trail was connected to the nearby Ghost Town Trail (see page 217) in Black Lick, Pennsylvania, forming a completed route of 46 miles between Indiana and Ebensburg. From Black Lick west to Blairsville a signed 8-mile on-road route connects to the West Penn Trail (see page 343), a 16-mile rail-trail that runs from Blairsville to Saltsburg.

A detailed brochure of the three trails is available from Indiana County Parks.

DIRECTIONS

To reach the Floodway Park trailhead in Homer City, located 5 miles south of Indiana, from State Route 119, turn onto State Route 56 West. Turn right onto Main Street in Homer City and continue to Floodway Park. A parking area is on the right. Park amenities include restrooms (closed during winter months), a pavilion, picnic tables and a playground. The trailhead is left of the parking lot.

To the Red Barn Trailhead in Homer City, from State Route 119, take Route 56 West in Homer City. Turn left on Main Street. Turn right on Kassal Street and continue to Red Barn Road. Turn right, then quickly left onto Boosters Drive. The Red Barn Access Area is on the right.

The north side of the trail above Homer City is wheelchair-accessible with a slight grade. The southern half of the trail has grades exceeding 5 percent.

Contact: Indiana County Parks and Trails
1128 Blue Spruce Road
Indiana, PA 15701
(724) 463-8636
www.indianacountyparks.org

Houtzdale Line Trail

T he old railroad line known as the Moshannon or the Mills branch crossed the Moshannon Valley during the mid- to late 1800s. The line was the foundation of the region's late 19th- and early 20th-century economy. The valley's vast reserves of coal were the object of the railroad expansion, and with the economically feasible transportation to industrial centers, mining boomed. The rail line carried sitting President Benjamin Harrison when he toured the coal fields in the surrounding area and addressed the citizens at the Houtzdale Station. The history of coal mining in the area is noticeable from the trail as it passes remnants of the industry. Interpretive signage along the trail commemorates significant historical structures and events.

Purchased from Conrail in 1994 following its disuse, the corridor was converted to a multi-use path to preserve the land as a public asset. The trail is lined with hedgerows of multi-flora and other deciduous shrubs.

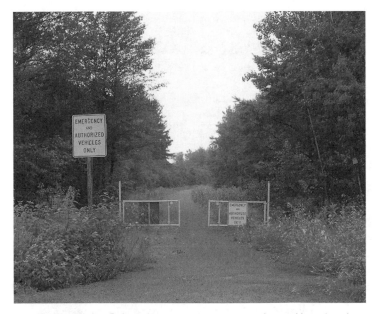

The Houtzdale Line Trail is tied to a rich coal-mining past, and as a rail line, it hosted President Benjamin Harrison on coal field tour.

Location
Clearfield County

Endpoints
Smoke Run to
Route 53/Coal Run
Road intersection in
Osceola Mills

Mileage
10.5

Roughness Index
2

Surface
Gravel

233

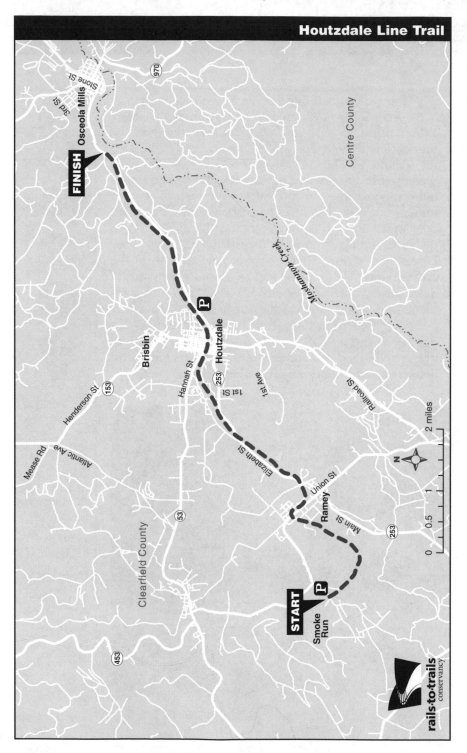

The entire length of the Houtzdale Line Trail is open for use with nearly 8 miles of improved surface from the Muddy Run Bridge west of State Route 2005 at Smoke Run to State Route 2007 just west of Osceola Mills. The trail has been graded, compacted and marked with mileposts. The extreme east and west ends of the trail remain in rough condition but are useable by hikers, mountain bikers and cross-country skiers. The best access point is at the trail center in Houtzdale.

Beyond Ramey and Houtzdale, the trail traverses natural areas of wetlands, upland forest and stream corridor with an abundance of wildlife and native plants.

DIRECTIONS

To reach the trail crossing in Houtzdale from Interstate 99, take 453 North to Viola and turn onto 153 North. (From Interstate 80 take the Clearfield exit for Route 879 South to 153 South). Park behind the BiLo Supermarket on Route 53 east of Houtzdale. On-street parking is available in Houtzdale and in Ramey on streets running parallel to the trail off State Route 453. A marked parking lot is now located off State Route 2005 in Smoke Run.

Contact: Houtzdale Line Rails to Trails Association
501 David Street
Houtzdale, PA 16651
(814) 378-7817
www.pawilds.com/explore/activity-details/index.
  aspx?id=222136

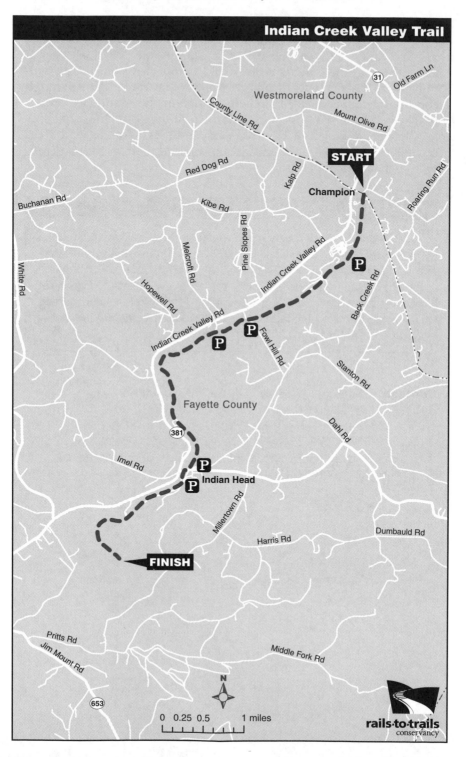

Indian Creek Valley Trail

O pen since 1989, the creekside Indian Creek Valley Trail traces the route of the Indian Creek
Valley Railroad (ICVRR), which was built early
in the 20th century. The rail line operated until 1926,
carrying passengers and freight between Indian Head
and Jones Mill, near the junction of Indian Creek and
the Youghiogheny River. The B&O Railroad bought the
ICVRR and operated the line until 1972. Then Western
Pennsylvania Conservancy acquired the corridor and
offered it to Saltlick Township.

Just north of Indian Head, you come to a cluster
of acid mine drainage remediation ponds, designed to
filter pollutants and sediment from water that passes
through the old mines. Around mile 3, the trail has numerous areas for picnicking and other outdoor activities. At about mile 4 the trail reaches the Melcroft Trestle, a pedestrian bridge that leads to a nearby park with
picnic tables and restrooms.

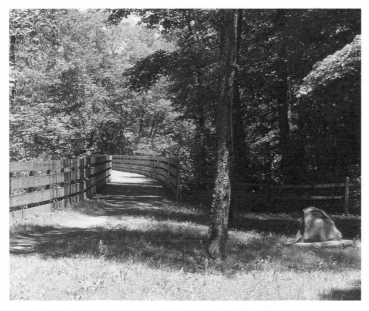

Parks and picnic areas line the path of the Indian Creek Valley Trail.

Location
Fayette County

Endpoints
Indian Head to
Champion

Mileage
6

**Roughness
Index**
1

Surface
Crushed limestone

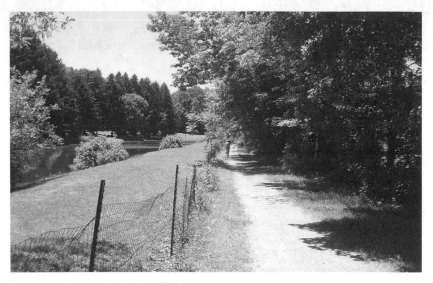

The trail runs along its namesake Indian Creek.

The trail appears to end at a street crossing in Indian Head, where there is another small park and a small general store. To continue on the trail, cross the street and follow the gravel road on the other side. In about a mile you will come to another segment of the trail, on your right as you head south. Horses and ATVs are prohibited on this trail.

DIRECTIONS

To reach the Champion Trailhead, take the Pennsylvania Turnpike to Exit 91 for Donegal. From the toll plaza, turn left onto Route 31 East and travel 2 miles. Turn right at Sarnelli's Market on Routes 381 and 711. Go about a mile to another stop sign, just before the Star Market. Turn left here onto County Line Road. Less than a quarter mile down County Line Road, cross a small bridge and you will see the trailhead marked.

Contact: Saltlick Township Municipal Building
P.O. Box 403
147 Municipal Building Road
Melcroft, PA 15462
www.visitpa.com/pa-maps/attraction-details/index.aspx?id=59686

Ironton Rail-Trail

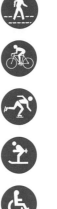

The Ironton Rail-Trail is the quintessential example of how a former rail corridor can transform a community. This trail has it all for locals and visitors alike. If you are looking for beautiful scenery, safe venues for exercise, and access to great parks and historical points of interest, you can't go wrong with this trail.

This corridor was originally the home of the Ironton Railroad, which began operating in 1860 with the primary purpose of transporting iron ore from the Ironton mines to the Lehigh Valley Railroad. As the iron ore industry dried up, the railroad continued to serve the local cement mills, until it fell into disuse in 1984.

The trail consists of a 6-mile loop and 3-mile spur. You can pick up the loop at Hokendauqua Park, a community park featuring parking, restrooms, a playground, baseball fields and basketball courts. This flat, paved section passes through wooded terrain and runs adjacent to Coplay Creek for a short section before turning north toward the town of Coplay where it runs past

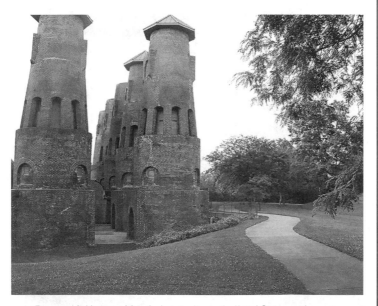

Two rows of old cement kilns, the last standing in the United States, are the must-see feature of the trail in Saylor Park.

Location
Lehigh County

Endpoints
Quarry Street
North in Whitehall
to Saylor Park
in Coplay

Mileage
9.2

**Roughness
Index**
1

Surface
Asphalt (loop) and
crushed stone (spur)

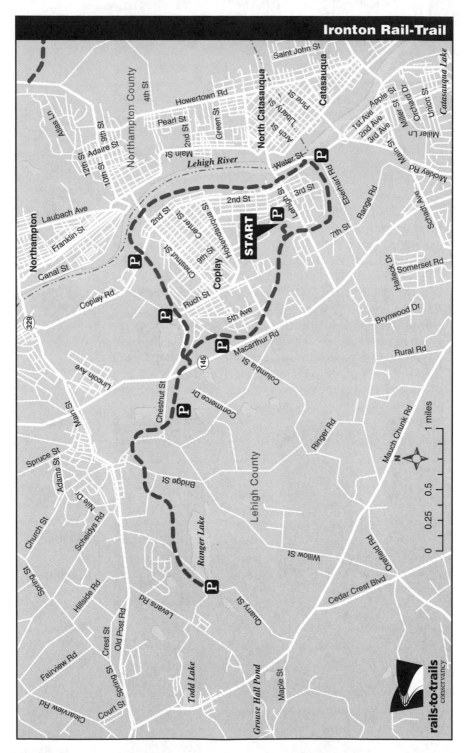

Ironton Rail-Trail

the Thomas Iron Works Property. Just after this property the trail is unfinished, and the surface changes to dirt before the paved surface picks up again at Saylor Park in Coplay.

With its two rows of beautiful old cement kilns reaching toward the sky, the last ones standing in the U.S., Saylor Park is a must-see. Don't miss the historical markers off the trail on the back side of the kilns that explains their relevance in American history. This small scenic park has a nice playground, open space for picnicking or sunbathing, and a parking lot.

About 2 miles past Saylor Park the trail loop intersects with the 3-mile spur. If you continue on the loop, you will travel through wooded areas and past neighborhood backyards before reconnecting with Hokendauqua Park.

The 3-mile spur has a crushed stone surface and offers a historical tour of the area's cement manufacturing heritage passing through scenic Whitehall Parkway with ruins of old buildings sprinkled throughout.

The trail ends on Quarry Road at another ample parking lot.

DIRECTIONS

To access the trail from Hokendauqua Park, take State Route 22 East to 145 North (Macarthur Road). Turn right on Lehigh Street and left onto Coplay Court. Immediately after going under the overpass, turn right into Hokendauqua Parking Lot.

To access the trail from Saylor Park, take 22 East to 145 North (Macarthur Road) but stay on 145 North. Pass Lehigh Street, and turn right onto Main Street. Turn right onto Coplay Road (bear right to stay on Coplay at the intersection with North Coplay) to Saylor Park.

To access the spur, take State Route 22 East to 145 North (Macarthur Road). Turn left on Mechanicsville Road. Turn right on Mauch Chunk Road and then turn right onto Quarry Street. You'll find the trailhead and parking lot on your left at the intersection of Quarry and Portland streets.

This trail is wheelchair-accessible.

Contact: Ironton Rail-Trail
c/o Whitehall Township
3219 MacArthur Road
Whitehall, PA 18052
(610) 437-5524
www.irontonrailtrail.org

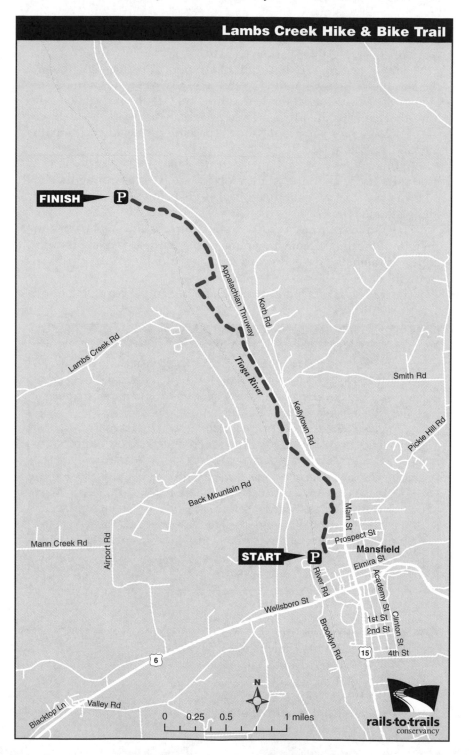

Lambs Creek Hike & Bike Trail

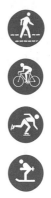

In 1979 the U.S. Army Corps of Engineers saw value in this corridor near the Tioga River, which was part of the Erie Lackawanna Rail Line. It once passed through the village of Lambs Creek, which is no more. The Corps paved the former rail line and created the Hike and Bike Trail. It still owns and maintains the trail today, with help from some local volunteers.

The trail heads from the town of Mansfield into the serene Pennsylvania countryside. It moves from openness near town into a thick growth of trees and brambles,

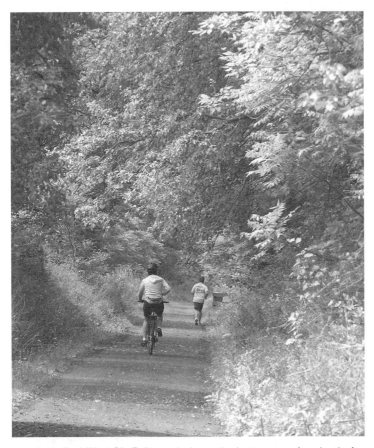

Lambs Creek Hike & Bike Trail is popular for exactly what its name implies; plus it's often used for local sports team training.

Location
Tioga County

Endpoints
Mansfield to
Lamb's Creek
Recreation Area

Mileage
3.5

**Roughness
Index**
1

Surface
Asphalt

making an appealing passage to explore and play. The trail has particularly lovely and distinct seasonal looks. Springtime showcases yellow-green willows in the wetlands; white and purple phlox drape the shoulders of the paved trail in the summer; and sumac bushes burn brilliant red and orange in autumn. Woodchucks and rabbits scamper across the trail with little concern for the human visitors, including the sports teams that use the trail for fitness training or the science classes out on field study.

While almost entirely flat with gentle curves, just outside town there is a surprisingly steep incline and dip to accommodate a terrain change. The farther from town, the quieter the trail becomes. Lambs Creek is visible from a few vantage points in the final mile of trail. Easy-to-follow signs make navigating the couple jogs in the route a cinch. The trail reaches its eastern terminus at the boat launch in the Lambs Creek Recreation Area. There are restrooms up the access road into the recreation area.

DIRECTIONS

To reach the Mansfield Trailhead, take US Route 15N (Business Route) to Mansfield (in town US 15 becomes Main Street). After the traffic light, cross Route 6 and go approximately four more blocks. Turn left on Corey Street, which takes you behind an IGA shopping center. Continue straight to the trail with parking on the left.

Contact: U.S. Army Corps of Engineers
R.R. 1, Box 65
Tioga, PA 16946
(570) 835-5281
www.nab.usace.army.mil/recreation/tioga.htm

Lebanon Valley Rail-Trail

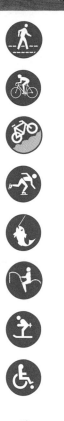

The Lebanon Valley Rail-Trail takes you on a journey into Pennsylvania Dutch country. Running along the corridor of the old Cornwall-Lebanon Railroad, the 14.5-mile trail lets you experience the beauty of farmland and forest, visit landmarks of the area's historical heritage, and sample the wide array of outdoor recreation that the region has to offer.

The railroad began operations in the 1880s and was built by Robert H. Coleman who received $1.2 million from the profits of Cornwall Furnace on his twenty-first birthday. The stock of the railroad was acquired by the Pennsylvania Railroad in 1913.

Well-maintained by volunteers, the trail features both a crushed stone path and a parallel equestrian path surfaced with dirt and wood chips. Proceeding south from the city of Lebanon, the trail shares a utility corridor until it passes under Zinns Mill Road. Rounding a bend, you'll come to the Cornwall Trailhead, which has adequate parking but no restrooms. The Cornwall Iron Furnace National Historic Site, remnants of a Revolutionary War–era iron foundry, is a short distance from the trail (www.cornwallironfurnace.org). The only charcoal cold blast iron furnace in the Western Hemisphere, the Cornwall Iron Furnace began operations in 1742 and was in use until 1883.

Just south of the furnace, the trail crosses a historic 130-foot iron-truss bridge. Here the trail begins a gentle climb and enters woodlands. Stay on the trail in this state game land area, and be aware of the dates of Pennsylvania hunting seasons. Near the top of the ridge, the trail shares a private drive for a quarter mile. This shared use is well marked. Once you reach the top of the ridge you are close to the village of Mount Gretna, a colorful town boasting Victorian cottages and a summer playhouse. Located on a wooded ridgetop, the Mount Gretna area is a popular destination for hikers, mountain bikers, canoers, kayakers and families coming to swim in Conewago Lake. It's worth hopping off the trail to visit the village, and perhaps get something to eat at

Location
Lancaster and
Lebanon counties

Endpoints
Zinns Mill Road in
Lebanon to Lebanon
and Lancaster
County line

Mileage
14.5

**Roughness
Index**
2

Surface
Crushed stone

245

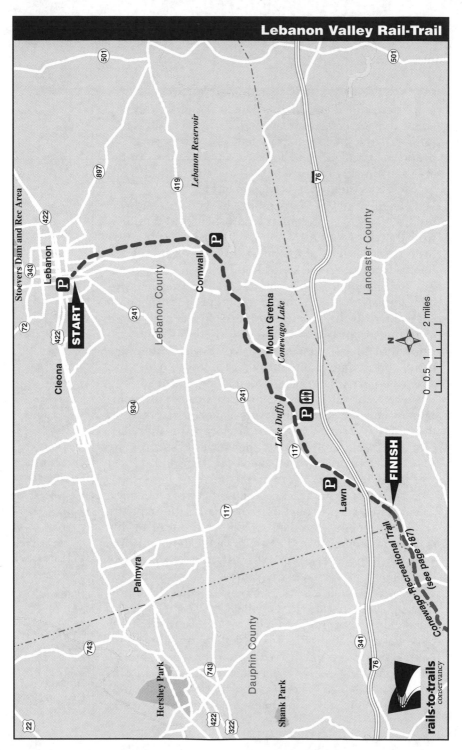

one of the area restaurants or browse through the craft shops. The Mt. Gretna Theater produces performances during June and July. A connecting trail, Mount Greta Spur, will take you into the village (www. mtgretna.com).

Beyond Mount Gretna, the Lebanon Valley trail slips through woodlands on a gentle downgrade to the Colebrook Trailhead. South of Colebrook, the trail moves into fields surrounded by farms. The Horseshoe Trail, used by hikers, equestrians and mountain bikers, intersects the Lebanon Valley trail about a mile south of the Colebrook Trailhead. The Lebanon Valley trail continues through rich Lebanon County farmland to the village of Lawn, where you can stop and browse small retail businesses. Another small trailhead provides trail access here, too. The trail continues through farmland and past horse farms to the Lancaster County line, where it joins the 5.1-mile Conewago Recreational Trail (see page 187).

DIRECTIONS

To reach the city of Lebanon Trailhead, take State Route 72 North from US Route 322. Turn right at Oak Street. Proceed two blocks and turn right on 8th Street. The trailhead is on your right near the intersection with Poplar Street.

To reach the Cornwall Trailhead, from US Route 322 in Cornwall, turn onto Boyd Street, which becomes Cornwall Road. Turn left onto Freeman Drive (State Route 419). The trailhead is on the left.

Contact: Lebanon Valley Rails-to-Trails
P.O. Box 2043
Cleona, PA 17042
(717) 867-2101
www.lvrailtrail.com

Lehigh Canal: North (D&L Trail)

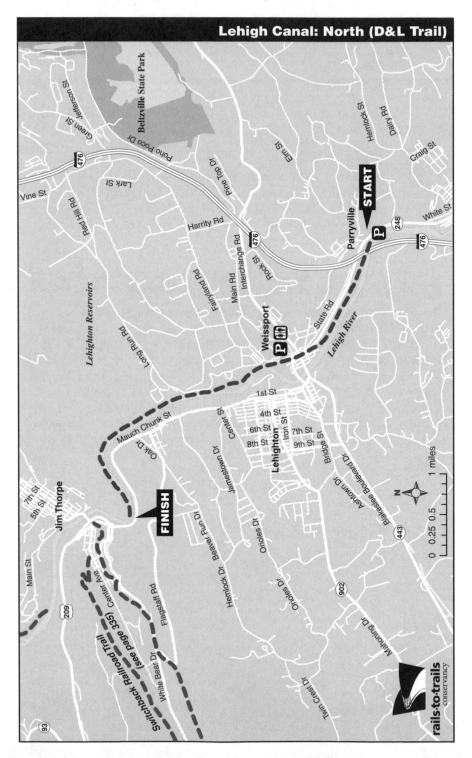

rails-to-trails
conservancy

Lehigh Canal: North (D&L Trail)

Josiah White, a famous entrepreneur and innovator, built the Lehigh Canal to transport anthracite coal the 46 miles from Mauch Chunk to Easton. There, the coal barges entered the Delaware Canal to complete their journey to Philadelphia. An ambitious feat of engineering, the Lehigh Canal used 44 locks and 8 dams to conquer the 353-foot elevation change. Remnants of these locks and dams can still be seen from the trail. Today, the canal is part of a larger national park known as the Delaware and Lehigh National Heritage Corridor. The Lehigh Canal: North (D&L Trail) traces the canal route from Parryville about 8 miles north to Jim Thorpe. Other rail-trails in close proximity include the Switchback Railroad Trail (see page 335) and the Lehigh Gorge State Park Trail (see page 255).

Starting from the small trail parking lot at the southern end of the trail in Parryville, you will find a narrow trail with a hard packed dirt surface. The trail runs next to active railroad tracks in Parryville for about 1.5 miles. After mile 1, stay on the right side of the trail (next to the canal) of a long commercial parking lot. Pick up the trail again at the northern end. From there the trail runs along the Lehigh River for another mile, and then follows the active tracks as they bend away from the river and lead you under Route 209 into Weissport where you will find another parking lot.

Once in Weissport, the trail improves dramatically. There is a pleasant signed trailhead with public parking and a picnic area. Be prepared for hoards of ducks to follow you if you stop for a picnic. The trail surface widens and is crushed stone from here on out. The ride is scenic with canal views on your right and built-in observation points as you cross each lock and dam. The left-hand side of the trail affords views of the Lehigh River, and wildlife such as beavers, minks, deer and waterfowl are common sights along the canal and riverbanks. The last mile winds down as the trail turns west and ends at a commercial site just outside of Jim Thorpe. There is no trail parking at this northern trailhead.

Location
Carbon and Northampton counties

Endpoints
Parryville to Jim Thorpe

Mileage
7.7

Roughness Index
1

Surface
Crushed stone and dirt

DIRECTIONS

To reach the Parryville trailhead, take Interstate 476 to Exit 74 to State Route 209. Follow 209 South to the traffic light just before the Lehigh River Bridge. Turn left here onto 248 South. Continue 1.7 miles to a trail parking lot on your right. Follow the dirt path south out of the parking lot and past the sign. Cross a small pedestrian bridge to get to the trailhead.

To reach the midpoint trailhead in Weissport, take Interstate 476 to Exit 74 to 209. Follow 209 South to the traffic light just before the Lehigh River Bridge. Turn right at the light onto Canal Street. Go a quarter mile, and turn left on Bridge Street when Canal Street dead-ends into it. The parking lot will be on your right immediately after you turn onto Bridge Street.

There is no access from the northern point.

This trail is wheelchair-accessible from Weissport northward.

Contact: Lehigh Canal Recreation Commission
P.O. Box 85
Ashfield, PA 18212
(610) 377-3856
www.delawareandlehigh.org

Lehigh Canal: South (D&L Trail)

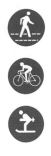

I f you feel like a stroll down the lazy river, then this is the trail for you. This peaceful trail follows the canal and Delaware River for almost its entire length. This trail offers a variety of path surfaces—wide paved asphalt, wide crushed stone and single-track packed dirt. And its meandering route through the trees makes it delightful. You'll likely see lots of geese and ducks, along with some canoes and kayaks, in the canal.

The 150-mile Delaware and Lehigh Canal Navigation System, built from 1817 to 1845, brought anthracite coal from the east central portion of Pennsylvania to various parts of the East Coast. With the building of the canal, several canal towns sprang up. There is interesting history along this trail: Easton hosted one of only three public readings of the Declaration of Independence, and during colonial times, the Liberty Bell rested secretly in Allentown. In the future, all 150 miles of the canal system, from Wilkes-Barre to Bristol, will be converted to trail.

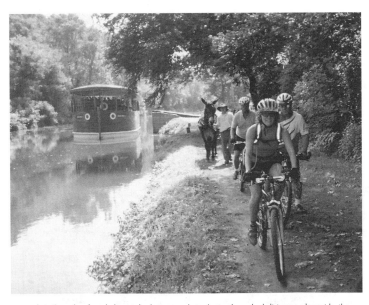

A trail made of asphalt, crushed stone and single-track packed dirt runs alongside the canal, allowing users to enjoy the lazy river atmosphere.

Location
Carbon, Lehigh and Northampton counties

Endpoints
Allentown to Easton

Mileage
13

Roughness Index
1

Surface
Crushed stone, dirt and asphalt

251

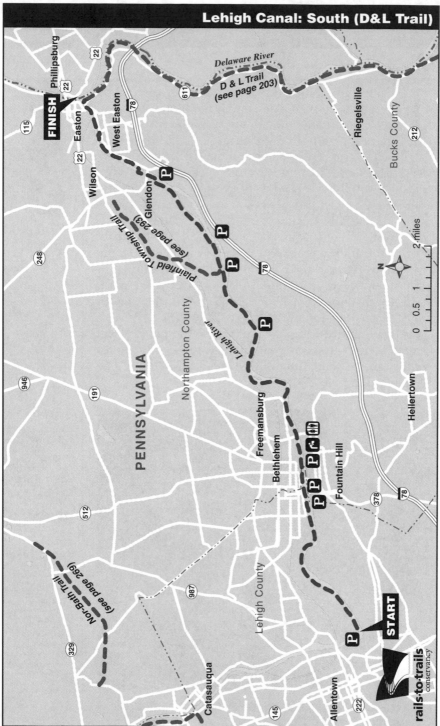

Lehigh Canal: South (D&L Trail)

DIRECTIONS

To access the trail in Allentown, take U.S. 22 East and exit at Airport Road. Follow Airport Road south for about 2 miles, until it becomes Irving Street. Follow Irving Street 1.25 miles to Hanover Avenue. Go right on Hanover, which becomes Hamilton Street. Turn right onto Albert Street. At the stop sign, turn right, cross the railroad tracks, bear left, and follow the canal through a small railroad underpass. Turn right at the fork, then immediately left on the other side of the canal. Follow to a small parking area and entrance to the trail.

To access the trail from Easton, take U.S. 22 to the 25th Street South exit to Lehigh Drive, turn right and go a half mile to the stop sign. Turn right and cross the old green Glendon Bridge. Then go right and follow the signs to the trailhead and picnic area.

Contact: D&L National Heritage Corridor
1 South Third Street, 8th Floor
Easton, PA 18042
(610) 923-3548
www.delawareandlehigh.org

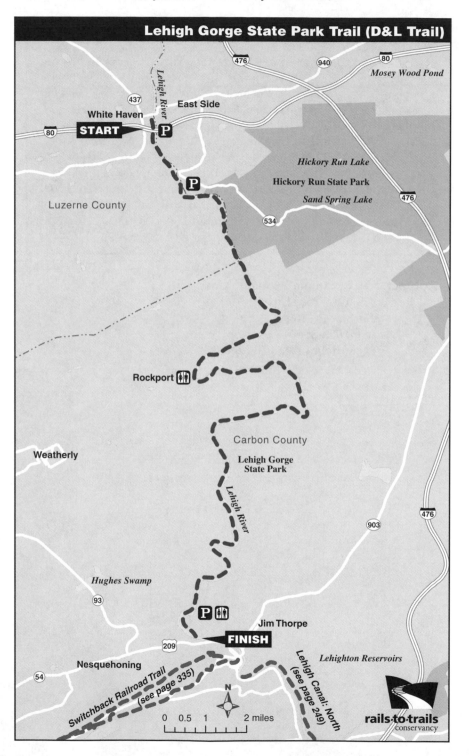

Lehigh Gorge State Park Trail (D&L Trail)

Lehigh Gorge State Park Trail (D&L Trail)

W hen coal was discovered in Summit Hill in the late 1700s a rush of development ensued in the Lehigh Valley. Josiah White and the Lehigh Coal and Navigation Company constructed a series of dams and canals in the early 1800s, to move coal to the markets down south. The canal system was wiped out by flooding in the mid-1800s, and the railroads took their place serving a booming logging industry. Fire ripped through the area and wiped out the logging industry in the late 1800s. The area became a tourist attraction until fire again swept through the region in the early 1900s, after which the gorge was abandoned. The Commonwealth of Pennsylvania began reclaiming the land in the 1970s.

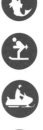

Today, thanks to their efforts, you will find one of the finest rail-trails for a wilderness getaway. This 26-mile trail cuts through 4,500 acres of dramatic river gorge parkland along the Lehigh River. Grab your bike

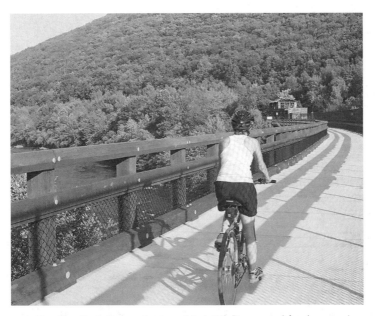

Along the entire route, you enjoy views of the Lehigh River on your left and occasional waterfalls on your right.

Location
Carbon and Luzerne counties

Endpoints
White Haven to Jim Thorpe

Mileage
26

Roughness Index
1

Surface
Crushed stone

255

and board a shuttle in Jim Thorpe to cycle from the northern point in White Haven to the southern point in Jim Thorpe. Or, if you are looking for a shorter, 15-mile experience, pick up the trail in Rockport.

Along the entire route, you enjoy views of the Lehigh River on your left and occasional waterfalls on your right. Although there is plenty of wildlife within the park, it isn't usually evident on the trail because the steep rock face on the right-hand side makes the trail difficult to reach from inland. However, herons and beavers are common wildlife to spot on the river side and you also might encounter an occasional snake or lizard. This 26-mile trail is certainly the highlight, but Lehigh Gorge State Park also offers opportunities to whitewater raft, fish, hunt and cross-country ski. The first 15 miles of the northern section is open to snowmobiling in winter months. Check the website for seasonal restrictions.

Although there is no obvious grade, cyclists do have to pedal to keep moving. During the last 5 miles of the trip, the trail runs next to an active railroad line that is elevated about three feet above the trail by a stone wall. Just 1.5 miles north of Jim Thorpe, the trail comes to a parking lot, then continues on, following the main road out to the recently renovated iron railroad bridge that crosses the Lehigh River. The bridge supports bicycle and pedestrian users, as well as an active railroad. An awesome reminder of the trail's origins, the bridge was

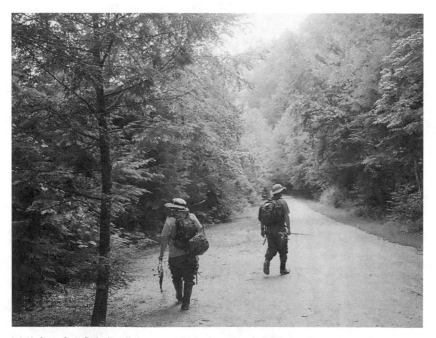

Lehigh Gorge State Park also offers opportunities to whitewater raft, fish, hunt and cross-country ski.

completed in 2009 after years of planning and provides an extra mile of trail leading into downtown Jim Thorpe.

The community of Jim Thorpe is a treat. Chock-full of charming shops, restaurants and inns, it has several outdoor outfitters that rent bikes and offer shuttles to the surrounding trails. Two other rail-trails to visit in the area are the Lehigh Canal: North (or D&L Trail, see page 249) and the Switchback Railroad Trail (see page 335). The shuttle ride costs about $16 per person.

DIRECTIONS

To reach the northern trailhead in White Haven, take Exit 273 from Interstate 80 into White Haven Borough. Follow State Route 940 east to the White Haven Shopping Center. Go through the shopping center parking lot and bear left to the state park access area.

To reach the southern trailhead just outside Jim Thorpe, from Interstate 476 take Exit 74 to 209 South. Follow State Route 209 out of Jim Thorpe to State Route 903 north, and cross over the Lehigh River to Coalport Road. Turn off of Coalport to Glen Onoko. Interestingly, 209 South actually runs north into Jim Thorpe, so don't be confused by that.

To reach the Rockport Trailhead (15 miles north of Jim Thorpe) from Jim Thorpe, take 209 South to State Route 93 north. Continue to Lehigh Gorge Drive into the village of Rockport. Turn on State Route 4014 to access the parking lot for this trailhead.

This entire trail is wheelchair-accessible.

Contact: Lehigh Gorge State Park
c/o Hickory Run State Park
RR #1, Box 81
White Haven, PA 18661
(570) 443-0400
www.dcnr.state.pa.us/stateparks/parks/lehighgorge.aspx

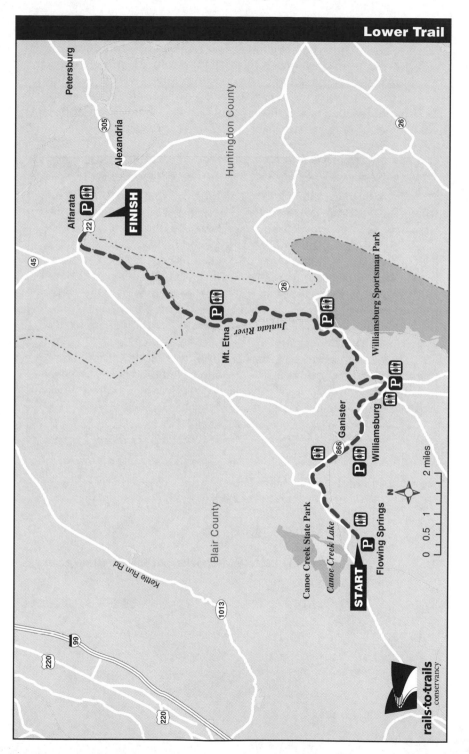

Lower Trail

G rab your bike or your walking shoes or saddle up your horse, and head for the cool breezes and dappled shade of the 17-mile Lower Trail. The name "Lower," which rhymes with "flower," refers to attorney T. Dean Lower, who provided the funds (one dollar) for the local rails-to-trails group to purchase the corridor in 1990 and create the trail.

The trail follows the Juniata River like a streamer in the breeze—at times crossing it, sometimes stretching out as if a gust of wind caught it for a few moments, but never straying far. The well-maintained, crushed limestone surface and nearly flat terrain makes travel an easy and pleasant effort. The scenery makes it a delight. Native trees of butternut, oak and bald cypress, among others, create a deep shade for most of the way, interspersed with farmland for short periods.

It glances through the heart of the communities of Point View, Ganister, Cove Dale and Williamsburg

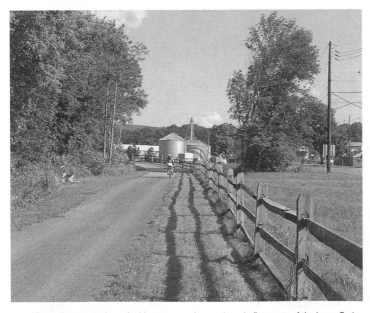

The well-maintained, crushed limestone surface and nearly flat terrain of the Lower Trail makes travel easy and pleasant.

Location
Huntingdon and Blair counties

Endpoints
Flowing Springs Road in Canoe Creek to Alfarata

Mileage
17

Roughness Index
1

Surface
Crushed limestone

259

along the way, like its predecessor: the Petersburg Branch of the Pennsylvania Railroad, which operated from 1879 to 1979. However the history of this corridor goes back even farther, to the 1830s, when it was part of the old Pennsylvania Canal—a system of waterways connecting Philadelphia to Pittsburgh used to transport goods on barges pulled by mules down the slow-moving canal and through numerous locks. Some of the canal locks and channels, as well as remnants of the lock tenders' houses, peek out from the thick vegetation if you look closely between Cove Dale and Mt. Etna and north of Williamsburg. Several times you pass over the Juniata River on re-purposed railroad bridges.

This peaceful trail is sheltered from the roads not far from its view. If you make your way quietly, or pause on a streamside bench or in one of the numerous covered shelters, you may be treated to seeing some of the furry creatures who live there—deer, rabbits, squirrels, turtles, black bears, turkeys, bobcats and more. In May trail users report seeing many species of migrating birds passing through the area—be on the lookout for bald eagles, great blue herons, ospreys, red-eyed vireos, cerulean warblers and scarlet tanagers, to name a few. The wildflower and the scenery change with each season, making it worth coming back time and again.

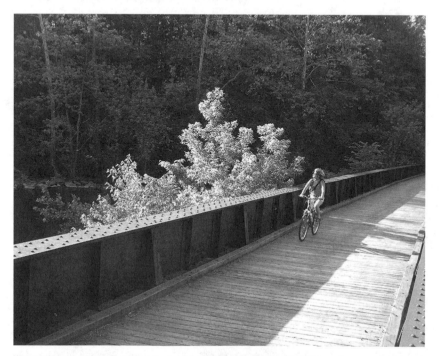

You may see some of the furry creatures that live along the trail. Plus the wildflowers and scenery change with each season.

DIRECTIONS

To reach the southern trailhead east of Hollidaysburg, start from Interstate 99 and US 220 to Exit 23 for Hollidaysburg, US 22E, Portage and Roaring Spring. Follow US 22 east for 8.2 miles. Pass Canoe Creek State Park on the left and turn right onto Flowing Springs Road. Cross the bridge and continue a mile to the parking area and trailhead on the left.

To reach the northern trailhead at Alfarata, follow US 22 to Alfarata. Turn north (left if coming from the west) onto Main Street just before the metal bridge. The parking is less than a quarter mile ahead on the right, and the trailhead is at the far end of the parking area.

There are trailheads with parking, picnic pavilions and chemical toilets at Ganister, Williamsburg, Cove Dale and Mt. Etna off of US 22.

To start the trail at Ganister Station, take US 22 from Hollidaysburg past Flowing Springs Road to turning east (right) on State Route 866. The trailhead and parking lot are to the right just after crossing the metal bridge.

The Williamsburg Station is reached by following State Route 866 past Ganister to Williamsburg. You come into town on West 1st Street, and go two blocks past the stop sign. Turn left onto High Street and into the parking lot and trailhead.

To reach the Cove Dale Station off of US 22, turn right (east) on Yellow Spring Road and then left on Cross Valley Road. Turn right at Fox Run Road, and then left onto Overlook Drive to the trailhead.

From Hollidaysburg to the Mt. Etna Trailhead, turn right (east) on Polecat Hollow Road and left on Fox Run Road. Turn right into the parking lot.

Contact: Rails to Trails of Central Pennsylvania
P.O. Box 592
Hollidaysburg, PA 16648
(814) 832-2400
www.rttcpa.org

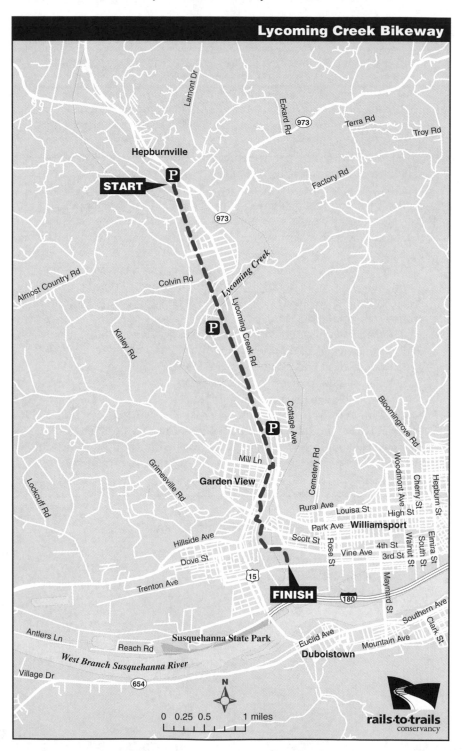

Lycoming Creek Bikeway

Lycoming Creek Bikeway

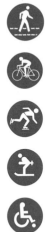

In a pretty valley between the West Branch of the Susquehanna River and Bald Eagle Mountain, the Lycoming Creek Bikeway is a fitting hometown asset. Tourists are not flocking to it, but the local folks have embraced it for their walks, morning run, ride with the grandkids, or an off-road route to one of several ballparks located just off the trail. The bikeway moves quite effortlessly from the rural hamlet of Hepburnville, south through the suburb of Garden View, and then arriving in Williamsport. A town of 30,000, the latter is recognized as a timber capital, but made famous as the home of Little League in 1939, and later for hosting the Little League World Series.

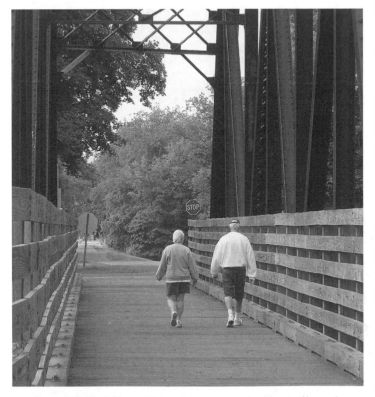

The Lycoming Creek Bikeway follows a straight course and passes smoothly over the winding Lycoming River several times using old railroad bridges.

Location
Lycoming County

Endpoints
Hepburnville to West 3rd Street in Williamsport

Mileage
5.5

Roughness Index
1

Surface
Asphalt

263

Native Americans used this pathway, which they called the Lagahani Trail, as part of a major transportation route between central Pennsylvania and the towns of Corning and Elmira, New York. Later Penn Central built a rail line on the corridor. In 1991 five area municipalities came together to develop the rail-trail.

Today its past is reflected in the straight course it takes, passing smoothly over the winding Lycoming River several times using old railroad bridges—including a 1901-vintage steel beauty at mile 1.7.

The northern end of the trail starts in trees at a community park on Bair Road in Hepburnville, and quickly opens up to farmlands with fields of corn and grasses and foraging rabbits. Most of the rest of the way is in open space where you can see the wide valley walls on both sides and ahead in the distance. Baseball fields are plentiful, and include the Carl E. Stotz Memorial Park, featuring a memorial to the Little League founder, and the Historic Bowman Baseball Park, the oldest minor league baseball stadium in Pennsylvania. Parking is available at the parks when a game is not in progress.

The trail runs beside Heshbon Park with sports fields and playground equipment (mile 1.8), which has parking. At mile 3.7, the trail takes a slight jog and parallels US 15 for a short distance before dipping under it. This segment of the bike path ends at Memorial Drive but you can catch the trail again by taking a left on Memorial Drive, going over the bridge and turning right to the trail. At mile 4.75 the

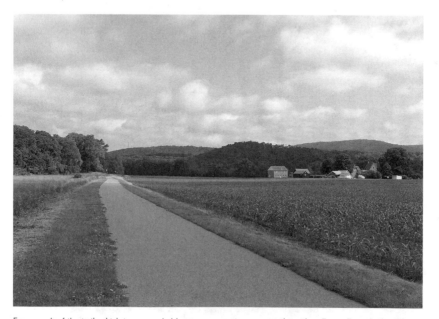

From much of the trail, which is surrounded by open space, you can see the wide valley walls on both sides and ahead in the distance.

trail comes to a bridge over Lycoming Creek. Cross the bridge, turn right, and come around on the far side of the river to pick up the trail again. It is up on a levee here, overlooking the river.

Another old railroad bridge across the creek graces the southern end of the bikeway at West 3rd Street in Williamsport, not far from US 15. It is open for traffic, though the trail does not officially cross the bridge here. If you want to continue from here, do so on-road.

DIRECTIONS

To reach the northern trailhead in Hepburnville, take US 15 North from Williamsport toward Mansfield. Take the exit for Beautys Run Road (State Route 29) going east (right) and turn left on Lycoming Creek Road, or 973. Turn left at Bair Drive, which leads into the Bair Community Park. Park in the lot on the left. The trail is past the parking at the end of the road.

To reach the Heshbon Park Trailhead, about 1.5 miles south of Bair Community Park, take US 15 North from Williamsport toward Mansfield. Take the exit for Beautys Run Road (State Route 29) and go right. At Lycoming Creek Road, turn right. Go about a half mile. Just after crossing the river, turn right on Log Run Road, which becomes Heshbon Road. In 0.4 mile, take a left into Heshbon Park.

To reach the Bowman Baseball Park Trailhead, from Interstate 180, take Exit 28 and turn right on Maynard Street. Turn left at West 4th Street (PA 2014), and continue about 8 blocks to the baseball park. Parking is also available at Historic Bowman Baseball Park.

Contact: Lycoming County Planning Commission
Lycoming County Courthouse
48 West Third Street
Williamsport, PA 17701
(570) 320-2138
www.lyco.org/dotnetnuke/Home.aspx

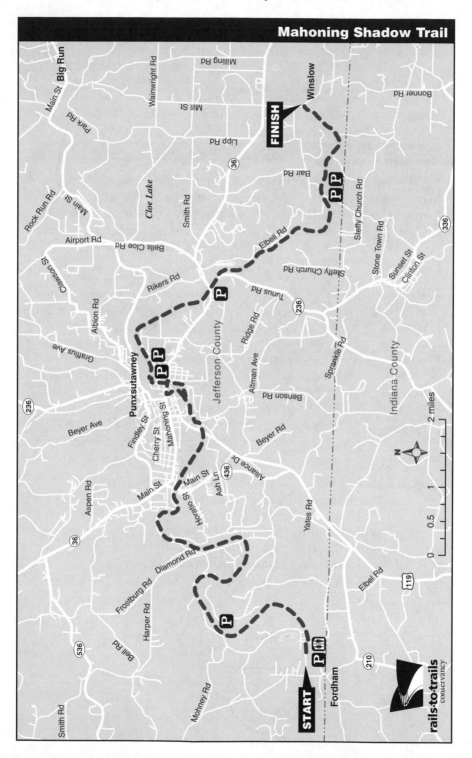

Mahoning Shadow Trail

Mahoning Shadow Trail

The Mahoning Shadow Trail has a flat surface that is easy for biking, running and walking. There is little signage on the trail, but each trailhead and access point is well marked.

Begin at the Fordham Trailhead. The trail parallels Mahoning Creek for several miles, then winds through the town of Punxsutawney. The trail surface is mostly crushed stone, dirt and on-street riding in Punxsutawney.

In Punxsutawney the trail is on-road for about a half mile to a skateboard park and baseball field at the end of Elk Street on the east side of town. From here, the trail winds through a thick wooded area to the small village of Cloe, then on to Winslow where the trail ends. (From the skateboard park to the Winslow Trailhead, there is a slight uphill grade).

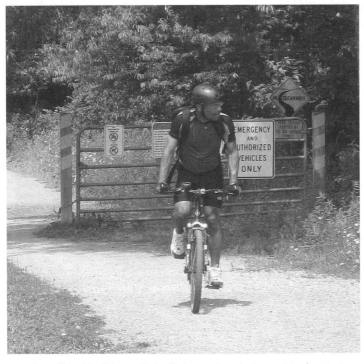

The surface of the Mahoning Shadow Trail is mostly crushed stone, dirt and on-street riding in Punxsutawney.

Location
Jefferson County

Endpoints
Fordham to Winslow

Mileage
15

Roughness Index
1

Surface
Crushed stone and dirt

When you are in Punxsutawney, stroll through the town square, get a quick bite to eat, or enjoy one of the town's many outdoor festivals.

DIRECTIONS

To reach the Fordham Trailhead, from downtown Punxsutawney, take Route 119 South. Follow Route 210 South as it turns right. Stay straight on Valier Road, or State Route 4025. Drive 0.8 mile and make a right at Center Street in Valier. Go 0.3 mile. A trail parking area will be on your right.

To reach the Winslow Trailhead, from downtown Punxsutawney, take Route 36 South for about 5 miles. Make a right on Winslow Road, toward Johnsonburg, then travel 0.6 mile on Winslow Road. Trail parking is on the right side of Winslow Road.

Contact: Punxsutawney Area Rails-to-Trails Conservancy
P.O. Box 16
Punxsutawney, PA 15767
(800) 752-7445
www.punxsutawney.com/trail/

Nor-Bath Trail

For 77 years, the tiny Northhampton & Bath Railroad traveled the 7 miles between the two Pennsylvania towns that gave the line its name. Then, like its larger cousins, the Northampton & Bath Railroad fell victim to the changing face of transportation and the rise of the trucking industry. After it fell into disuse in 1979, the corridor was purchased by Northampton County, thus allowing the "little train that could" to continue to serve its namesake towns by connecting their parks, schools and historic centers.

Today you'll find a pretty, tree-lined, crushed stone trail that is perfect for a walk or ride. Starting in a residential area of Northampton, the trail soon emerges into rural terrain that features open fields, bubbling streams and pretty little bridges. At mile 2.5 you reach the perimeter of Bicentennial Park. Here you'll find 64 acres of county parks with restrooms, pavilions, playgrounds,

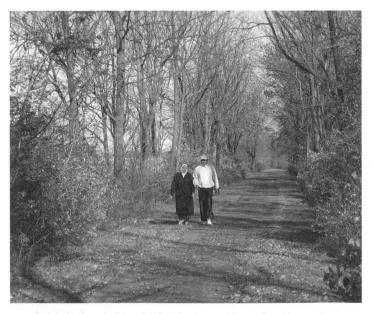

The tree-lined, crushed stone Nor-Bath Trail is perfect for a walk or ride.

Location
Northampton County

Endpoints
Northampton to Bath

Mileage
4.5

Roughness Index
1

Surface
Crushed stone

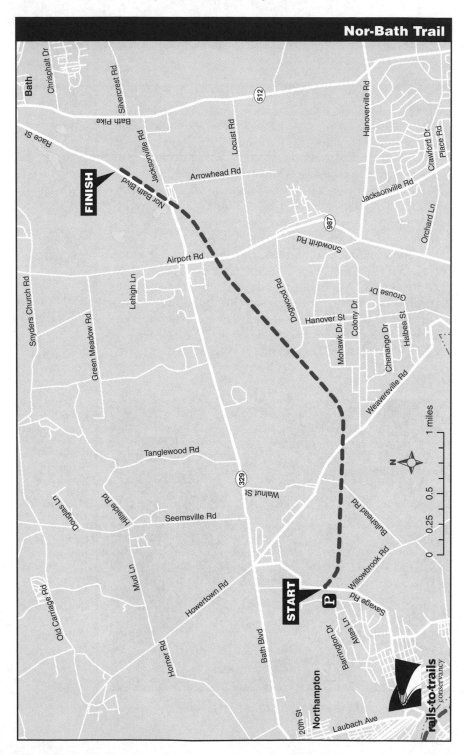

Nor-Bath Trail

tennis courts and a wide variety of ball fields. You can enter the park via a short access trail between miles 2.5 and 3.

Along the way several street crossings, well-designed for safety, require you to maneuver through a fenced turnstile and dismount from your bike. Wildlife is abundant along the way—from chipmunks dodging in and out of your path to the occasional rabbits that also claim the trail as home.

The trail winds down with beautiful views of farmland before crossing Jacksonville Road. Currently the trail goes only a short distance farther to end at State Route 987 near a cement factory. Eventually the trail will extend another mile into Bath.

Pets are prohibited on this trail, unusual for a rail-trail.

DIRECTIONS

To reach the Northampton Trailhead, take State Route 987 North out of Allentown to 329 West. Turn left on Howarton Road (you'll see Howarton ballpark at the intersection). Bear right onto Atlas Street then left on Savage Road. You'll find a small parking lot on the left at the signed trailhead.

The trail is also accessible from Bicentennial Park in Northampton, which has ample parking. The trailhead outside of Bath ends on State Route 987 near the intersection with Jacksonville Road. There is no parking available.

This trail is wheelchair-accessible.

Contact: Northampton County Parks and Recreation
R.D. 4, Greystone Buidling
Nazareth, PA 18064
(610) 746-1975
www.dcnr.state.pa.us/

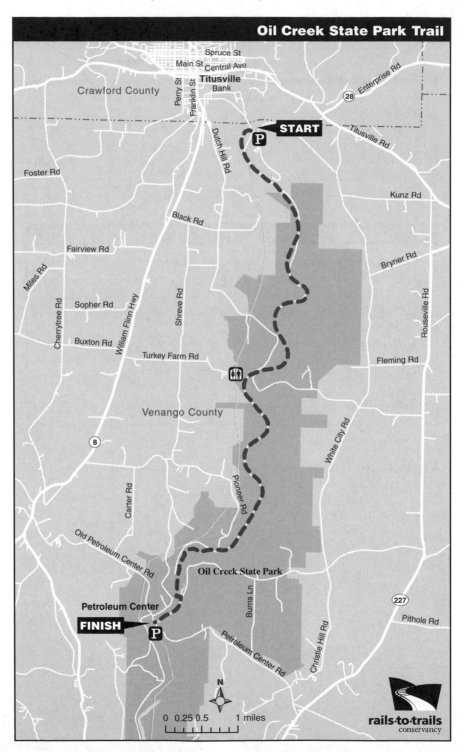

Oil Creek State Park Trail

Spruce St
Main St
Central Ave
Titusville
Bank
Perry St
Franklin St

Crawford County

Enterprise Rd

28

Dutch Hill Rd

START

P

Titusville Rd

Foster Rd

Kunz Rd

Black Rd

Fairview Rd

Bryner Rd

Miles Rd

Cherrytree Rd

Sopher Rd

Shreve Rd

Buxton Rd

William Flinn Hwy

Rouseville Rd

Turkey Farm Rd

Fleming Rd

P

Venango County

8

White City Rd

Carter Rd

Pioneer Rd

Old Petroleum Center Rd

Oil Creek State Park

Burns Ln

227

Petroleum Center

Pithole Rd

FINISH

P

Christie Hill Rd

Petroleum Center Rd

N

0 0.25 0.5   1 miles

rails·to·trails
conservancy

Oil Creek State Park Trail

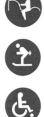

The Titusville and Petroleum Center Railroad had one major purpose when it was built in 1863—to transport oil. Oil was discovered in Oil Creek Valley in 1859 by Colonel Edward Drake and William Smith. Almost overnight, towns such as Titusville, Miller Farm, Pioneer and Petroleum Center blossomed as opportunists rushed to get rich from the Great Oil Dorado. The oil boom ended in 1871 almost as quickly as it began. When the once-boisterous towns died, the railroad hung on. Through a series of mergers, it became part of the Pennsylvania Railroad system in 1900 and fell into disuse in 1945. Connecting routes for bicycle and pedestrian use

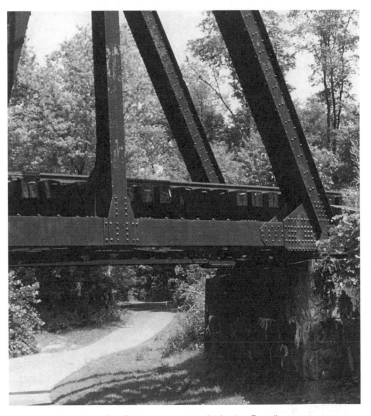

The Oil Creek State Park Trail runs beneath the Oil Creek & Titusville excursion train, known locally as the OC & T.

Location
Crawford and Venango counties

Endpoints
Crawford and Venango County line south of Titusville to Petroleum Center

Mileage
9.7

Roughness Index
1

Surface
Asphalt

273

between Oil Creek State Park and the Samuel Justus Trail (see page 305) were signed and completed in 2010.

Few reminders of the thousands of people who once occupied the Oil Creek Valley remain. Today, the valley is home to hemlocks, beaver ponds, trout streams (outstanding fly-fishing) and waterfalls. The only evidence of the intense oil drilling that once went on here is the occasional well head.

The Oil Creek Trail has a flat, easy surface and is suitable for users of every level. Nearby Oil Creek State Park has 52 miles of hiking trails with camping shelters and 20 miles of cross-country ski trails. Picnicking, canoeing, fishing, bicycle rentals and other facilities, such as restrooms, food and lodging are available in the nearby town of Titusville. The Oil Creek & Titusville excursion train, known locally as the OC & T, runs through the park. Stay awhile and take a train ride back 150 years into the heart of the country's first oil fields. Every August the Oil Festival arts and crafts show offers lots of fun, food, and unique sights that highlight the area's history and local culture.

DIRECTIONS

For the south trailhead, take the Route 8 bypass north around Oil City and continue 3 miles. Turn toward Petroleum Center on State Route 1007 just after Route 8 crosses Oil Creek. Continue 3 miles to the junction of State Route 1007 and State Route 1004. Turn right on State Route 1004 and cross Oil Creek. Parking is 0.1 mile ahead on the left.

For the northern trailhead at Drake Well Museum, take the Route 8 bypass around Oil City, and proceed 14.4 miles north along Route 8. Turn right at the light on Bloss Street. If you reach the junction with Route 27 you have passed Bloss Street. Continue a little more than 0.75 mile to trailhead parking on the right before the bridge.

Contact: Oil Creek State Park
305 State Park Road
Oil City, PA 16301
(814) 676-5915
www.dcnr.state.pa.us/stateparks/parks/oilcreek.aspx

Palmer Township Recreation Trail

The Palmer Township Recreation Trail (formerly the Towpath Bike Trail) is a terrific community asset for Palmer and Bethlehem township residents and a great destination for visitors as well. Three modes of transportation once operated on this corridor: Lehigh Canal, the Central Railroad of New Jersey and the Lehigh Valley Transit (LVT) interurban. Chartered in 1818, the privately owned canal remained in operation for 113 years, hauling anthracite coal from Mauch Chunk to the Delaware Canal at Easton. The Easton and Western branch was built in 1914 and fell into disuse in 1972. The LVT Easton line was part of a larger electric railways system that stretched from the Delaware Water Gap to near Philadelphia.

Today a smooth, 8-foot-wide asphalt trail traverses the corridor in a partial loop running 8 miles from Easton High School to Riverview Park. The 7-mile loop is the heart of the trail. The small spur section running south from Easton Area High School in Palmer Township makes a nice connection for locals to access the trail. The spur section that runs north from the high school has been closed.

Mostly tree-shaded, the trail is very pretty and well maintained, with mile markers, benches and flowerbeds

Location
Northampton County

Endpoints
Palmer Township
to Bethlehem

Mileage
7.8

Roughness Index
1

Surface
Asphalt

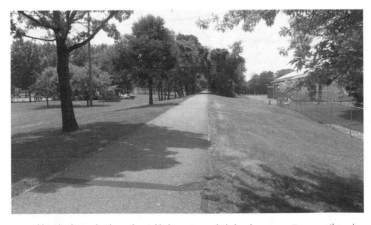

After the first mile, the path quickly becomes secluded and serene as it weaves through farmland and woodland.

275

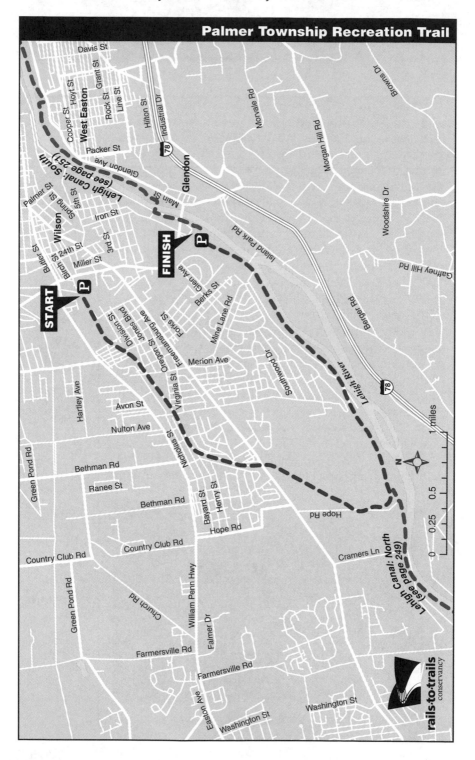

Palmer Township Recreation Trail

sprinkled throughout. Starting at the high school, you cruise down a gentle grade to Riverview Park, which lines the banks of the Lehigh River. The first mile of trail passes through neighborhoods and parks, but the path quickly becomes secluded and serene as it weaves through farmland and woodland.

Around mile 5 the trail starts to loop back and runs along the river, although at this point the distance and tree cover make river views hard to see. Close to mile 6 the trail intersects with another rail-trail the Lehigh Canal: South (or D&L Trail, page 251), which heads south to Allentown. To stay on the towpath trail and complete the loop, bear left. At this point, you start to see the river off to your right, and as you glide along the next to the river, stop and enjoy the gorgeous Chain Dam overlook. As the trail comes to a close you wind back from the water's edge through Riverview Park, with its picnic areas, ball fields, pavilions, restrooms and parking. Fishing is also available at this park.

To extend your sightseeing, take the short distance (on road) out of the parking lot down Lehigh Drive, and turn right to go over the Glendon Bridge into Hugh Moore Park. This great recreational park offers canal rides on boats drawn by horses plying the old towpath, historical markers sharing the canal's history, and open green space to picnic, play soccer or relax.

DIRECTIONS

To reach the Riverview Park Trailhead, from Allentown, take US Route 22 East to 25th Street South. Stay on 25th Street South for about 2 miles, and turn right on Lehigh Drive. Turn right into the parking lot.

To reach the northern trailhead, from Allentown, take US 22 East to 25th Street South. Turn right onto William Penn Highway (Easton Avenue). Almost immediately you will see a shopping center on your right and Easton High just beyond it. Turn left onto 27th Street, which dead-ends at the entrance to the trail. A small gravel area here does *not* have posted parking restrictions.

This trail is wheelchair-accessible.

Contact: Palmer Township Board of Supervisors
P.O. Box 3039
Palmer, PA 18043
(610) 253-7191
www.palmertwp.com/boards/recreation/bikepath/
   BikePathMap.pdf

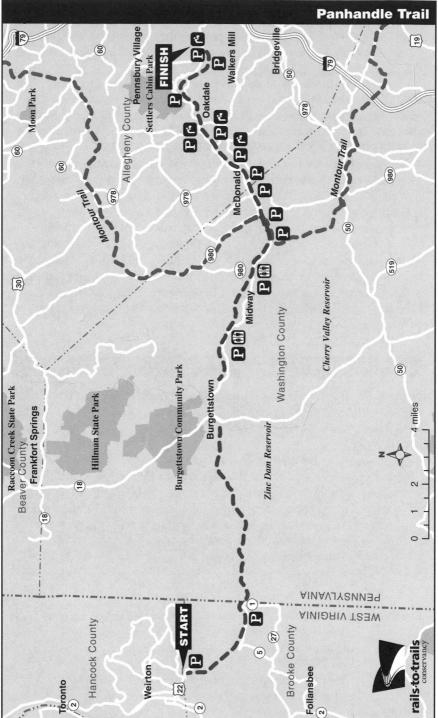

Panhandle Trail

Panhandle Trail

The Panhandle Trail is another jewel in the Pittsburgh metro area trail system. A Conrail line, known as the Panhandle Railroad, once connected Pittsburgh to Cincinnati, Chicago and St. Louis on this route. The rail corridor has been transformed into a multi-use, non-motorized trail stretching 29 miles, from Weirton, West Virginia, to Carnegie, Pennsylvania.

Today, the wide trail is open to pedestrians, cyclists and horseback riders, with many easy access points along the way. Locals have created colorful sculptures out of recycled materials, such as handcrafted birdhouses, and colorful old shoes, to enhance the trail. You never know what art you may come across.

Spring and summer, when flowering shrubs and wildflowers dress up various landscaped trailheads and access points, are great times to bike the Panhandle.

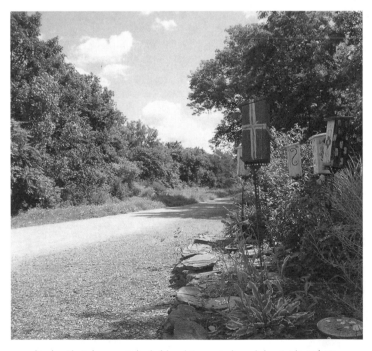

Local residents have created colorful sculptures out of recycled materials, such as handcrafted birdhouses and colorful old shoes, to enhance the trail.

Location
Allegheny, Brooke and Washington counties

Endpoints
Weirton, West Virginia, to Carnegie, Pennsylvania,

Mileage
29

Roughness Index
1

Surface
Crushed stone

Between June and October, the Collier Friends of the Panhandle Trail sponsors several annual events on the trail. The friends group also maintains the trail from Walkers Mill to Greg Station.

The Panhandle Trail connects to the Montour Trail between the village of Primrose and town of McDonald and will eventually link to Washington, D.C., via the Great Allegheny Passage (see page 221). Recognized as a valuable resource and landmark for residents, the Panhandle Trail was the 100th successful rail-trail project in Pennsylvania. Officials from Washington and Alleghany counties, the West Virginia Rail Authority, PennDot, the U.S. Surface Transportation Board, the Pennsylvania Department of National Resources, and the Southwestern Pennsylvania Commission continue to work to preserve the historic corridor and develop the trail.

DIRECTIONS

To reach the Carnegie Trailhead, take Interstate 79 South to Noblestown Road. Turn and head west 1.7 miles to Walkers Mill. Turn left on Walkers Mill Road, and then go 0.1 mile to a parking lot on the right where the trailhead is marked.

To reach the Montour and Panhandle trails Trailhead near Champion, West Virginia, follow State Route 22 West from Pittsburgh to 980 South just west of Champion. Take State Route 980 South to McDonald, and turn right on State Route 4012. Continue on 4012 to the village of Primrose. The trailhead parking and access is at the intersection of John's Street and Noblestown Road.

Contact: Panhandle Trail Association
807 Timber Trail
Oakdale, PA 15071
(724) 693-0870
www.panhandletrail.org

Path of the Flood Trail

Though it memorializes a sad occasion, the Path of the Flood Trail is a beautiful, tranquil trail. In the Johnstown Flood of 1889, the South Fork Dam failed and more than 2,200 townspeople lost their lives. The first 2 miles of the trail opened in 2007, extending from the historic Staple Bend Tunnel, believed to be America's oldest railroad tunnel, and continuing on-road to a wooded hillside. This section ends at the Franklin Ball Field in Johnstown, where it connects to the Allegheny Portage Railroad Trail. It is part of the Mainline Canal greenway, and there are plans to extend the trail to the town of Ehrenfeld, southeast to Alleghany Portage National Park to Cresson. This extension would be part of the Mainline Trail, a rail-trail that was part of the Old Portage Railroad and the South Cambria Trolley Line.

The 2-mile Path of the Flood Trail is hilly in some sections, as it follows a portion of the Little Conemaugh

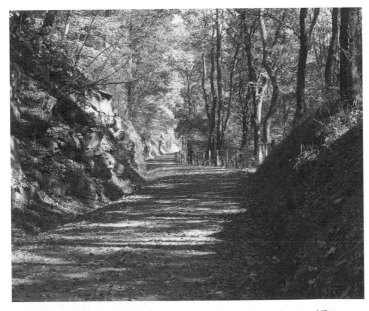

The Path of the Flood Trail is heavily canopied with large trees, and native wildflowers flourish throughout the section leading from the tunnel to Franklin Ball Field.

Location
Cambria County

Endpoints
Ehrenfeld Park to the Staple Bend Tunnel, Franklin Ball Field

Mileage
2

Roughness Index
2

Surface
Asphalt and ballast

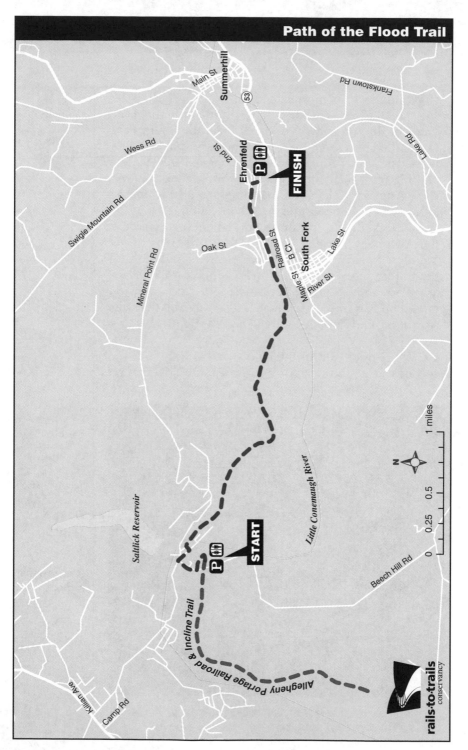

Path of the Flood Trail

River. Mostly ballast, with asphalt near the tunnel, the trail is used mainly by joggers, walkers and cross-country skiers.

A few memorial markers relating to the flood are posted along the trail. While in the area, you may want to poke around the Johnstown and Cambria County area, where several 1860s-era buildings from the area's steel industry prime are being restored to their former glory.

During the summer months, the trail is heavily canopied with large trees, and native wildflowers flourish throughout the section leading from the tunnel to Franklin Ball Field. Benches along the trail overlook an active rail-line and a lush green valley.

DIRECTIONS

To the tunnel trailhead, from the Johnstown National Memorial, follow US 219 North to State Route 53 North, Railroad Street. Exit toward South Fork and Portage, and turn right on State Route 53 to Summerhill. Turn left on Main Street, then turn right on Madison Street, and turn left on Jackson Street. Go approximately 1 mile on Jackson Street, which becomes Swigle Mountain Road (State Route 3043). Bear left onto Mineral Point Road. Use caution on the steep hill.

Turn left on Beech Hill Road and proceed over the bridge to the railroad underpass. Drive under the underpass and up the short hill. The trailhead is on the right, marked by a large sign and nicely landscaped with an informational kiosk at the far end of the asphalt parking lot.

Contact: Cambria County Parks and Recreation Authority
401 Candlelight Drive, Suite 234
Ebensburg, PA
(814) 472-2110
www.co.cambria.pa.us

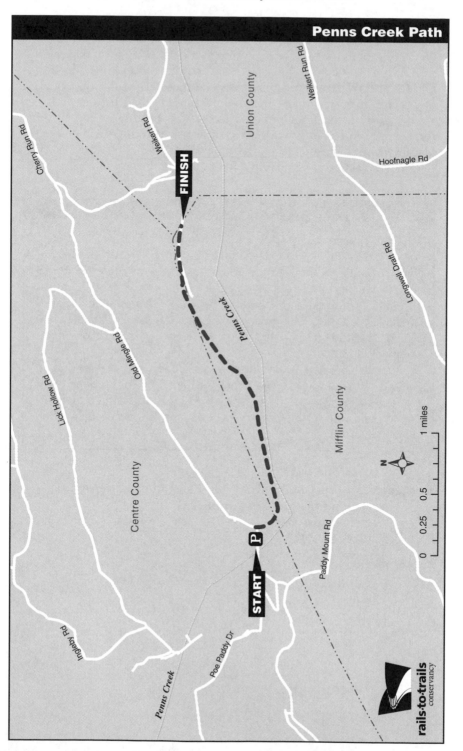

Penns Creek Path

Though little-known compared to other popular rail-trails in Pennsylvania, the Penns Creek Path is worth the effort of visiting for a scenic bike ride or hike in the forest. Pretty in all seasons, it is especially picturesque in June when its mountain laurel bushes abound with beautiful white blossoms.

The trail forms part of the Mid-State Trail, a 319-mile cross-country hiking trail that traverses five state forests and eight natural areas in the ridge and valley region of central Pennsylvania; with its firm surface, the Penns Creek Path is more suitable for cycling than most other sections. Penns Creek Path is tucked away in Poe Paddy State Park at Poe Mills, a former lumber town dating from the timber industry boom in the late 19th century. The trail follows the path of a small timber railroad that once threaded through this mountainous region to transport lumber to State College.

Starting out from the roadside trailhead near Poe Mills, you soon come to a narrow, rustic footbridge that

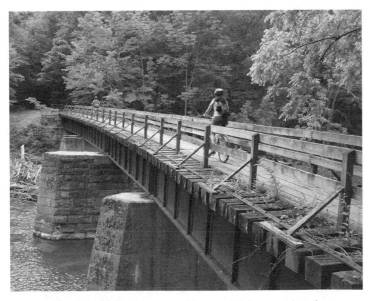

A narrow, rustic footbridge crosses Penn Creek near the beginning of the trail, and looking down you are likely to see people fly-fishing.

Location
Centre, Mifflin and Union counties

Endpoints
Poe Paddy State Park to Cherry Run

Mileage
3.6

Roughness Index
2

Surface
Ballast and stone dust

285

crosses Penns Creek. It's best to walk your bike across the bridge since the wood planks run lengthwise, leaving gaps that may catch bike tires. Look down to the water as you cross, and you are likely to see fly-fishermen hoping to snag a trout with the Green Drake fly (a fishing fly especially popular at Penns Creek in late May and early June).

Just beyond the bridge is the next thrill, a former railroad tunnel carved into the rock face. It curves just enough to block any light from the other end, making it pitch-black for a short distance inside. A headlight or flashlight makes it less creepy and helps you avoid stepping in the rubble spilling into the pathway from the inside walls.

Beyond the tunnel the trail delivers a serene woodland experience. At mile 1.5 Penns Creek becomes visible again through the foliage. From here to the end of the trail, larch and pine trees share space with the deciduous trees lacing the sky. The crushed stone surface gradually fills with equal amounts of grass, giving the impression of being less-traveled. Near the end of the trail at Cherry Run, the Mid-State Trail breaks off to the left heading uphill.

DIRECTIONS

To reach the Poe Mills Trailhead, take US 322 to Potters Mills and turn east (right if you are traveling north on US 322) on Decker Valley Road. Continue about 10 miles, following the signs to Poe Valley State Park. Stay on this road through Poe Valley State Park to Poe Paddy State Park (an additional 3 miles from Poe Valley State Park). Most of this route from US 322 is unpaved. Turn left into the park, cross a one-way bridge, stay straight, and continue about a half mile. On the right is a small sign for Penns Creek Path. Park beside the road.

Contact: Mid-State Trail Association
P.O. Box 167
Boalsburg, PA 16827
(410) 931-2946
http://hike-mst.org/

Perkiomen Trail

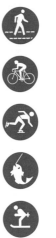

The history of Perkiomen Trail railroad corridor extends more than 140 years. Founded shortly after the Civil War, the Perkiomen Railway Company started running from Oaks to Pennsburg in 1868. New transportation spurred development along the line, which then extended to Emmaus and the Lehigh Valley. In the 1920s the Perkiomen Valley was a favored vacation spot, and people used the railroad for access to recreation areas. The Reading Company bought the line in 1944, but a decline in recreational interests, suburban development on natural lands, and the advent of the automobile as the favored form of transportation caused passenger trains on this route to cease operations by 1955.

Much of the old railroad right-of-way has been preserved as the Perkiomen Trail, a 19.5-mile multi-use trail

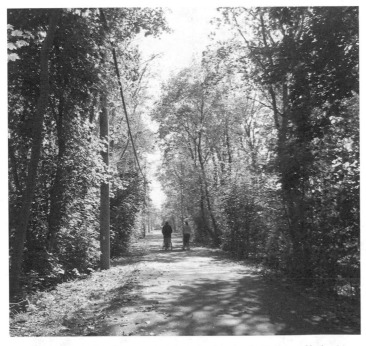

The trail travels through serene wooded areas and rural and suburban neighborhoods, providing an everyday escape, as well as a versatile community transportation route.

Location
Montgomery County

Endpoints
Green Lane
and Oaks

Mileage
19.5

Roughness Index
1

Surface
Crushed stone
and asphalt

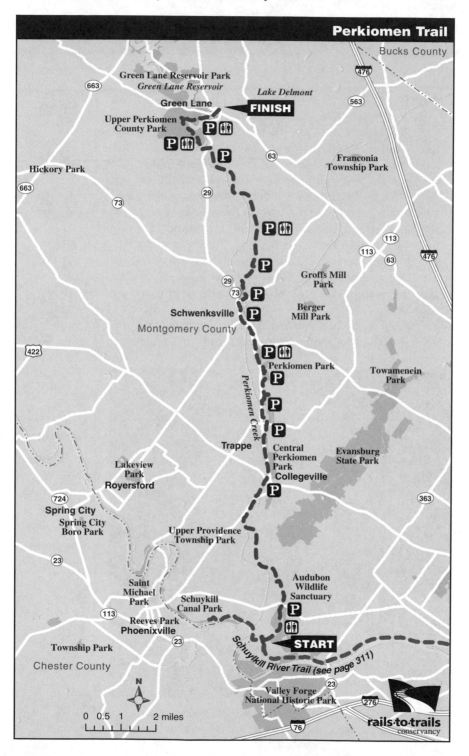

Perkiomen Trail

Bucks County

Green Lane Reservoir Park
Green Lane Reservoir

663

476

Lake Delmont

Green Lane   **FINISH**

563

Upper Perkiomen
County Park

P 🚻

P 🚻

P

63

Franconia
Township Park

Hickory Park

663

29

73

P 🚻

113

113

63

476

P

Groffs Mill
Park

29

73

P

Schwenksville

Montgomery County

P

Berger
Mill Park

Towamenein
Park

422

P 🚻

Perkiomen Creek

Perkiomen Park

P

P

P

Trappe

Central
Perkiomen
Park

Collegeville

Evansburg
State Park

Lakeview
Park

Royersford

P

363

724

Spring City

Spring City
Boro Park

23

Upper Providence
Township Park

Saint
Michael
Park

Schuykill
Canal Park

113

Reeves Park

Phoenixville

23

Audubon
Wildlife
Sanctuary

P

🚻

Township Park

Chester County

START

Schuylkill River Trail (see page 311)

N

Valley Forge
National Historic Park

23

0 0.5 1   2 miles

76

rails·to·trails
conservancy

276

extending from its connection with the Schuylkill River Trail in Oaks to Green Lane Park in Green Lane. The trail passes through a rich and varied landscape, including town centers, parks and rural areas, and parallels scenic Perkiomen Creek for much of its route. Most of the trail is surfaced with cinder and packed gravel, with some paved segments. The trail serves as a regional access between Green Lane Park in Green Lane, Central Perkiomen Valley Park in Schwenksville, and Lower Perkiomen Valley Park in Oaks, as well as two very significant sites, the Mill Grove Landmark in Audubon and Pennypacker Mills Site in Schwenksville.

The trail travels through serene wooded areas and rural and suburban neighborhoods, providing an everyday escape and also a versatile community transportation route. Small businesses along the trail demonstrate its immense popularity. One highlight comes near the southern end of the trail, right where the trail meets up with Schuylkill River Trail. Here you can experience Valley Forge National Historic Park. In addition to enjoying a wonderful visitor center, explore the grounds where George Washington and the Continental Army famously retreated to in the winter of 1777 to 1778.

DIRECTIONS

To reach the Oaks Trailhead, from the Pottstown Expressway (State Route 422), take the Egypt Road exit near Valley Forge National Historic Park. After exiting, head east on Egypt Road for a few hundred feet, and take your first right onto New Mill Road. Continue into the Lower Perkiomen Valley Park, where there is parking and trail access.

To reach the Green Lane Trailhead, follow 29 North past Schwenksville, and bear right in Zieglerville to follow 29 North to Perkiomenville. Go left on Dead Creek Road and continue a half mile to the trailhead in the county's Green Lane Park.

Contact: Montgomery County Department of Parks
& Heritage Services
P.O. Box 311
Norristown, PA 19404
(610) 278-3555
www.montcopa.org/parks/perkiomentrail/Perkiomen.htm

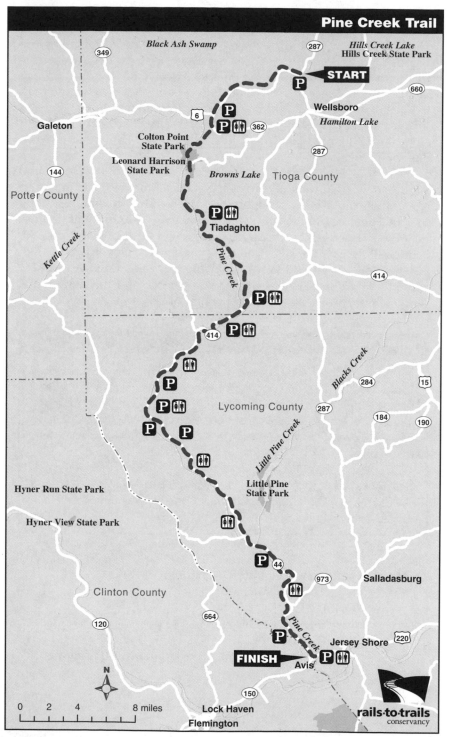

Pine Creek Trail

Black Ash Swamp

349

287

Hills Creek Lake
Hills Creek State Park

START

660

6

362

Wellsboro

Hamilton Lake

Galeton

Colton Point
State Park

Leonard Harrison
State Park

Browns Lake

287

Tioga County

144

Potter County

Pine Creek

Tiadaghton

414

Kettle Creek

414

Blacks Creek

284

15

Lycoming County

287

184

190

Little Pine Creek

Little Pine
State Park

Hyner Run State Park

Hyner View State Park

44

Salladasburg

973

Clinton County

Pine Creek

664

Jersey Shore

220

FINISH

Avis

120

N

150

Lock Haven

Flemington

0   2   4   8 miles

rails·to·trails
conservancy

Pine Creek Trail

One of the premier rail-trails in the Northeast, the Pine Creek Trail in Pine Creek Gorge offers travelers a spectacular, 62-mile journey through the area commonly referred to as the Grand Canyon of Pennsylvania. With numerous trailheads, comfort stations, campgrounds and small towns along the route, the well-maintained trail is ideal for an afternoon excursion, or a longer trek.

The Jersey Shore, Pine Creek & Buffalo Railroad began operating here in 1883, carrying timber to sawmills in towns along the floor of the gorge. The railroad also transported coal north to New York State. The last freight train passed through in October 1988.

Relatively flat, with a grade of only 2 percent, the trail runs from Ansonia south to Jersey Shore, traversing Tioga and Tiadaghton state forest lands. For 55 of its 62 miles, it hugs Pine Creek, providing great views of dramatic rock outcrops and numerous waterfalls, and

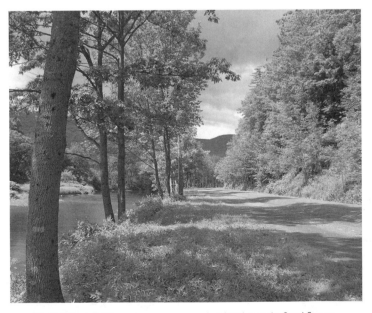

The Pine Creek Trail traverses an area commonly referred to as the Grand Canyon of Pennsylvania.

Location
Lycoming and Tioga counties

Endpoints
Ansonia to Jersey Shore

Mileage
62

Roughness Index
2

Surface
Crushed stone

access to whitewater rafting and canoeing in the spring. You may be lucky enough to see an eagle, osprey, coyote or even a black bear on the hillside adjacent to the trail. Other wildlife, including deer, wild turkeys, herons, hawks, river otters and beavers, also can be spotted in the gorge.

Horseback riding is allowed on portions of the trail. To use the hard-packed dirt path beside the trail between Ansonia and Tiadaghton, equestrians should park at the Ansonia Trailhead.

There are many other access points along the route. Several access points with parking are located south of Blackwell along Route 414. The parking lot at Rattlesnake Rock is a popular drop location for canoe and bicycle shuttle services. Another large parking lot is located at the southern end of the trail just north of Waterville. A trail map and detailed maps of the state forests are available at the Bureau of Forestry Offices in Wellsboro and in South Williamsport.

DIRECTIONS

To reach the northern trailhead, from US 6, where it meets PA 287 north of Wellsboro, turn left to travel north on PA 287 and then turn left on Patten Road. The trailhead is on the left beyond the ice cream shop.

The reach the southern trailhead, from US 220 in Jersey Shore, turn right or south on Thomas Street, travel three blocks and turn right onto Railroad Street. Travel eight blocks; the trailhead is on your left.

Contact: Tioga County Visitors Bureau
2053 Route 660
Wellsboro, PA 16901
(570) 724-0635
www.visittiogapa.com/railtrail.html

Tiadaghton State Forest
432 East Central Avenue
South Williamsport, PA 17702
(570) 327-3450

Plainfield Township Trail

From 1880 until well into the 20th century, Bangor and Portland Railway steam locomotives plied this corridor and others in the region, providing essential transportation services for the nearby quarries. Conrail bought the Plainfield Township Trail line in 1976, only to close it five years later. The township then bought the corridor and built the rail-trail.

A fine recreation destination for a variety of visitors, from walkers to mountain bikers, cross-country skiers and wheelchair users, the trail is well maintained and signed. Most of the pathway is surfaced with an unusual crushed red stone. Large trees line the trail on both sides, framing pretty views of Bushkill Creek as it meanders in and out of view. The trail crosses the creek five times, on charming wooden bridges. One on the southern end offers a particularly dramatic view of the creek far below. You can enter the trail at midpoint, or stop there for a rest; there is a parking area, picnic facilities and a trailhead.

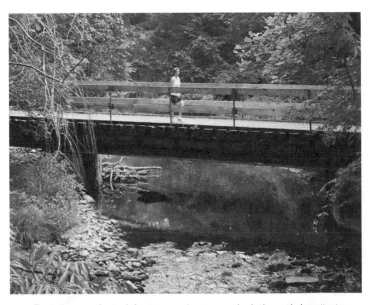

The trail crosses the creek five times on charming wooden bridges with dramatic views.

Location
Northampton County

Endpoints
Wind Gap to
Stockertown

Mileage
6.7

**Roughness
Index**
1

Surface
Crushed stone and
hard-packed dirt

293

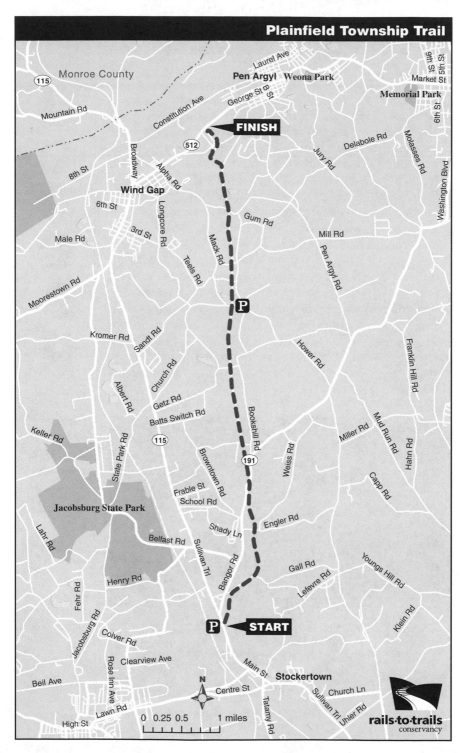

Plainfield Township Trail

This trail is actively used by horseback riders. Even if you don't see a horse on the trail, you will pass pretty farms and see horses grazing in the fields. Be alert, as the trail crosses several roads.

On the northern end, the trail crosses State Route 641. After this crossing, the trail surface changes to heavy ballast and is more difficult for cyclists. One mile farther up, the trail branches. Go right onto a narrow dirt pathway to Pen Argyl Road, or left up a steep grade that will level off quickly and wind around a working quarry. The quarry is fenced off for security, but you get a nice view all the same.

DIRECTIONS

To reach the southern trailhead in Stockertown, take the Stockertown exit off of Route 33 and turn right at the first stop sign. At the next light, turn left onto Sullivan Trail Road. Continue about 0.75 mile and pass a power station on the right. Park in the lot past the power station.

To reach the midpoint trailhead, travel south out of Wind Gap on 115 (South Broadway). Turn left on East 3rd Street. Make a right onto Church Road, then left on 633 Knitters Hill Road. The parking lot will be on your left.

There is no parking at the northern trailhead.

This trail is wheelchair-accessible with the exception of the section north of State Route 641.

Contact: Plainfield Township
6292 Sullivan Trail
Nazareth, PA 18064
(610) 759-6944
http://twp.plainfield.pa.us/recreation.html

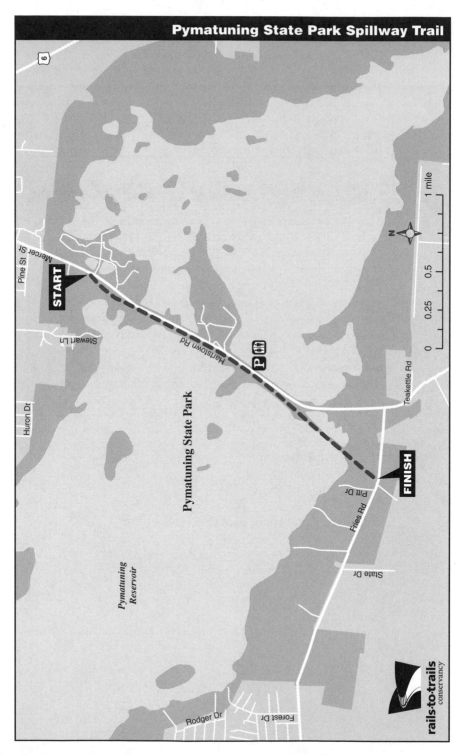

Pymatuning State Park
Spillway Trail

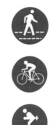

Located on the abandoned Erie and Pittsburgh branch of the Pennsylvania Railroad, this short but intriguing trail runs through Pymatuning State Park, a large and popular two-state recreation area encompassing a 2,500-acre wildlife refuge around Pymatuning Reservoir. (The word *Pymatuning* is derived from an Iroquois term, probably from the Seneca tribe, that means "crooked-mouthed man's dwelling place.")

Pymatuning State Park Spillway Trail, a beautiful 3-mile route adjacent to Linesville Road, crosses the Pymatuning Spillway, which was built in 1930. The Pymatuning Spillway is one of the most popular tourist attractions in the area; it is estimated that more than 300,000 visitors come to view the local beauty and feed bread to the numerous carp that gather around the spillway. The Pymatuning Spillway is known as the place

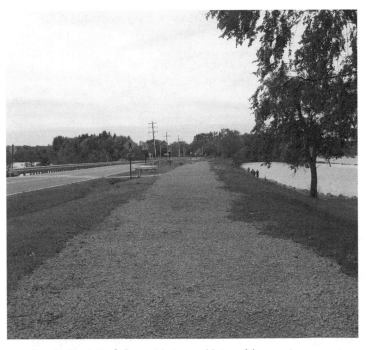

Cross the Pymatuning Spillway to take in peaceful views of the reservoir.

Location
Crawford County

Endpoints
Pymatuning
State Park

Mileage
2.9

Roughness Index
1

Surface
Ballast

where "ducks walk on fishes's backs." The area has plenty of attractions, including campgrounds, a fish hatchery and the Game Commission Wildlife Learing Center in the middle of the spillway.

DIRECTIONS

To reach the spillway trailhead, from Interstate 79 North, take Exit 147B for US 322 West and US 6 West toward Conneaut Lake. Merge onto Conneaut Lake Road and US 19, 322 and 6. Follow US 6 for a little more than 7 miles. Continue on PA 6 (Water Street) for another 6 miles and then turn left to stay on PA 6 as it turns left for a half mile to Linesville. Turn left on South Mercer Street, which turns into Hartstown Road and takes you directly onto the spillway after about a mile. Parking is available on spillway on your left and at other locations in the park.

Contact: Pymatuning State Park
2660 Williamsfield Road
Jamestown, PA 16134
(724) 932-3141
www.dcnr.state.pa.us/stateparks/parks/pymatuning.aspx

Radnor Trail

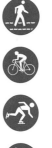

This 2.4-mile paved trail provides a quiet, scenic escape northwest of Philadelphia. The trail travels mostly through wooded areas, passes near local parks and is lined with several benches.

Founded in 1902, the Philadelphia and Western Railway Company (P&W) was intended to be part of Jay Gould's proposed intercontinental electric railway. Gould's grand and progressive plan was scaled back, as was the route of the P&W Trains, featuring luxurious, elaborately appointed cars, traveled from Philadelphia's 69th Street Station to suburban Strafford. For the first few months, the trains ran every quarter hour, with the full route taking a half hour. The line remained active until 1956, when it was replaced with bus service.

In 2005 Radnor Township celebrated the opening of the multi-purpose Radnor Trail. Running through residential areas, the trail provides a popular off-road route

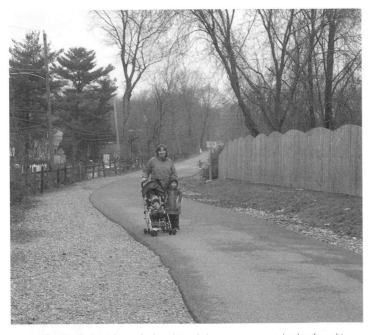

Location
Delaware County

Endpoints
Sugartown Road to Radnor Chester Road in Radnor

Mileage
2.4

Roughness Index
1

Surface
Asphalt

The Radnor Trail travels mostly through wooded areas, passes near local parks and is lined with several benches.

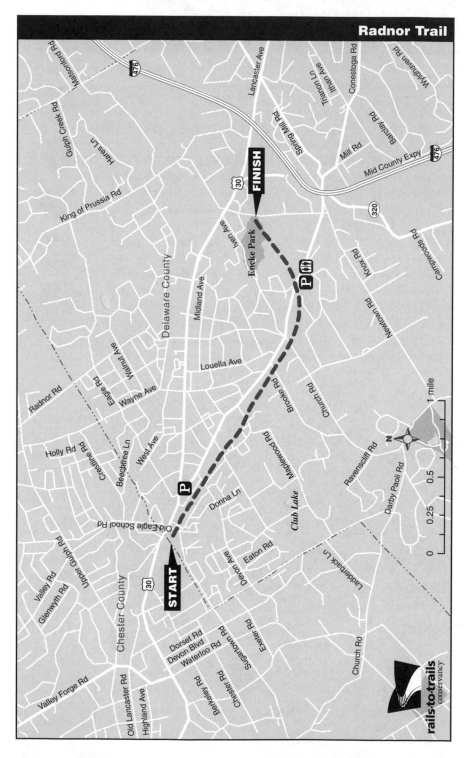

to retail centers and schools. The 2.4-mile trail runs from Encke Park at Radnor-Chester Road to the shopping center at Sugartown Road and Route 30.

DIRECTIONS

To reach the trailhead, from Interstate 476 take Exit 13 onto Route 30 west. Continue and turn left onto Radnor-Chester Road. Continue and turn right onto Conestoga Road. Proceed on Conestoga Road to trail parking on your left, near the intersection with Brookside Avenue.

This trail is wheelchair-accessible.

Contact: Radnor Township
301 Iven Avenue
Wayne, PA 19087
(610) 688-5600
www.friendsofradnortrails.org

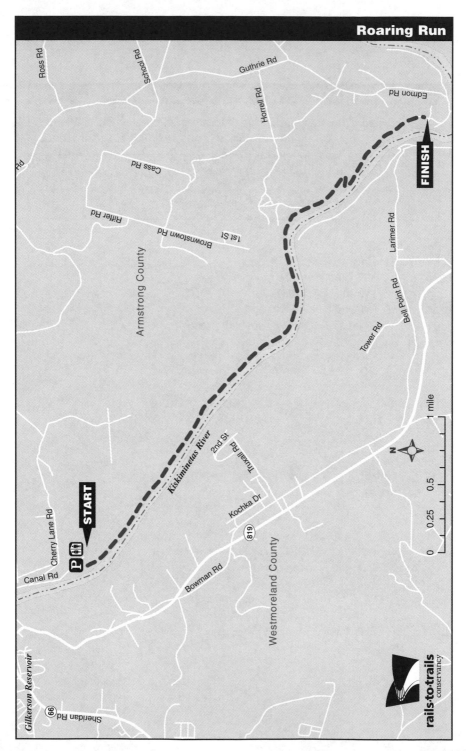

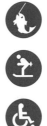

T he out-and-back Roaring Run is the third incarnation of this pathway. First to occupy the waterfront site was the Pennsylvania Main Line Canal towpath, which operated between 1825 and 1850. The Pennsylvania Railroad Apollo Industrial Track was eventually built on the unused towpath, and the trains carried coal from the Leechburg Coal mining station.

The Pennsylvania Railroad donated the right-of-way to Roaring Run Watershed Association, a group formed in 1982 to help preserve this historic area and clean up pollution from former mines. The group opened the trail in 1991.

Beginning at the parking area on Canal Road, Roaring Run parallels the Kiskiminetas River to the southeast. At mile 1.5, you can see the stone remains of canal Lock No. 15. A 16-foot-high dam once stood here; it was destroyed by a flood in 1866, but during low water some remnants are visible. The trail is in excellent condition and well maintained as it meanders next to the beautiful Kiski River. It will eventually connect to the West Penn Trail (see page 343) a mile downriver, creating a trail system from Ebensburg to Apollo.

DIRECTIONS

Take the Pennsylvania Turnpike to Exit 75 for New Stanton. Follow the turnpike Route 66 extension to its end in Delmont. Follow Route 66 North from Delmont to Apollo. After crossing the bridge in Apollo, turn right on Kiski Avenue. Follow Kiski Ave for 0.7 mile, which then turns into Canal Road. Proceed to the marked trailhead parking at the end of the road. This entire trail is wheelchair-accessible.

Location
Armstrong County

Endpoints
Canal Road in Kiskiminetas

Mileage
5

Roughness Index
1

Surface
Crushed limestone

Contact: Roaring Run Watershed Association
P.O. Box 333
Apollo, PA 15613
(724) 478-3366
www.roaringrun.org/Site/Home.html

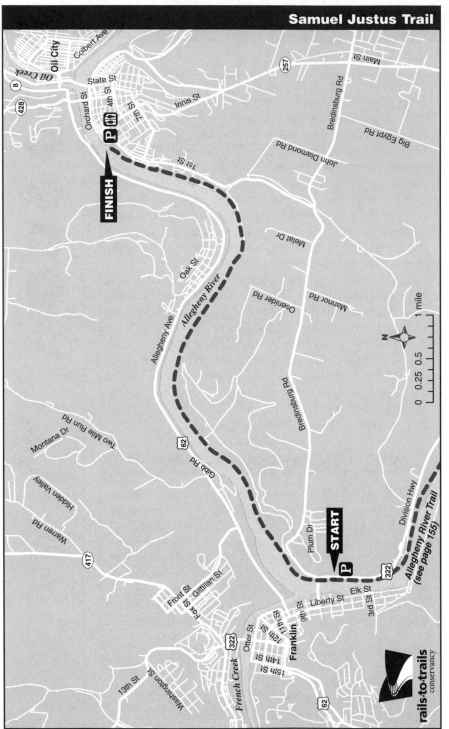

Samuel Justus Trail

Samuel Justus Trail

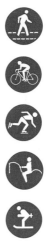

onnecting Oil City and Franklin, the Samuel Justus Trail is a 6-mile segment of a 30-mile trail following the former Allegheny Valley Railroad. The A.V. was completed to Oil City in 1868 and connected the oil fields with Pittsburgh. It operated as an independent company until it was absorbed into the Pennsylvania Railroad system in 1910. Conrail stopped using the line in 1984.

The trail begins across the Allegheny River from Franklin (where it also connects to the Allegheny River Trail, see page 155), known for its well-preserved Victorian architecture and tree-lined streets. It follows the river north toward Oil City through lush woodlands, passing iron furnaces, several operating oil wells, Pioneer Cemetery and a visitor center in an 1844 saltbox house. The trail's paved surface is perfect for bicycling

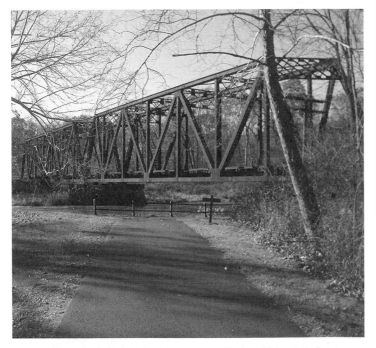

Location
Venango County

Endpoints
Franklin to Oil City

Mileage
6

Roughness Index
1

Surface
Asphalt

The Samuel Justus Trail is a 6-mile segment of a 30-mile trail following the former Allegheny Valley Railroad, a rail line that connected oil fields with Pittsburgh.

and inline skating. You may also want to visit the mansion of the late Senator Joseph Sibley, who made his fortune by inventing the first formula for refining crude oil.

DIRECTIONS

To access the trail in Oil City, follow Interstate 80 to Exit 29. Follow Route 8 North, crossing the intersection with Route 322, and continue to follow Route 8 (Route 62) to Oil City. Cross the Allegheny River on the Petroleum Street Bridge. Continue to the second light, and head right on West 1st Street. Continue about 1.5 miles to trailhead parking on the right, just past the Penelec building.

To access the trail in Franklin, follow Interstate 80 to Exit 29. Follow Route 8 North to Route 322. Follow 322 East (Liberty Street) through Franklin. After crossing the Allegheny River on the 8th Street Bridge, park at the trailhead on the right.

Contact: Allegheny Valley Trails Association
Box 264
Franklin, PA 16323
(814) 432-4476
www.avta-trails.org

Sandy Creek Trail

The Sandy Creek Trail carves its way through some of the most remote and spectacular countryside in northwestern Pennsylvania. This 12-mile paved trail has some impressive features, including tunnels and massive trestles like the Belmar Bridge, which crosses the mighty Allegheny River. This trail also connects to both the Allegheny River and Samuel Justus trails (see pages 155 and 305).

Beginning in the village of Van in the Clarion Highlands, this trail descends for the first 8 miles following Sandy Creek as it trickles down to the Allegheny River. Along this section, you cross numerous railroad trestles, some quite high with far-reaching views of the surrounding forests and hillsides. As you meander along the trail, you eventually reach the Sandy Creek Tunnel about a mile before hitting the Allegheny River. This former rail tunnel will cool you off on a warm summer day.

The trail eventually meets up with the Allegheny River, precisely where Sandy Creek empties out into it and where you can pick up the Allegheny River and

Location
Venango County

Endpoints
Van to Fisherman's
Cove near Franklin

Mileage
12

**Roughness
Index**
1

Surface
Asphalt

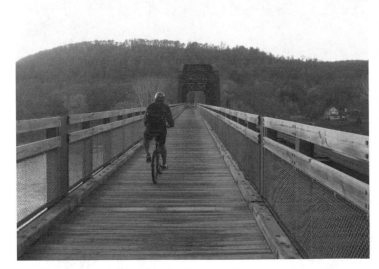

The trail crosses numerous railroad trestles, some with far-reaching views of the surrounding forests and hillsides.

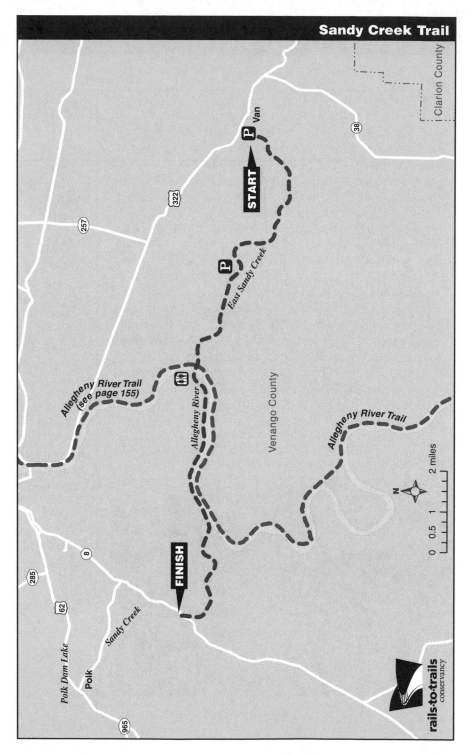

Samuel Justus trails. Before crossing the Belmar Bridge, look for the sign down to them. Both follow the eastern banks of the river.

The 1385-foot Belmar Bridge is a stunning example of the once booming railroad industry in the area. Originally built with funding from John D. Rockefeller, the bridge was intended to serve as a vital link on a corridor from New York to Chicago. In the end, the trestle and corridor were used more regularly to service the local coal industry. The trestle and trail cross the Allegheny River, where, after reaching the western bank, the trail turns left (southwest) and follows the river downstream.

The trail continues to follow the river's western shoreline for the remaining 4 miles. The gentle, wide river gives the area a soothing feeling like it has remained in this state for thousands of years. The trail eventually reaches its terminus near Fisherman's Cove, where there is a backcountry access road.

DIRECTIONS

To reach the Van Trailhead, follow 322 South/East out of Franklin and continue until you reach the village of Van. Take a right onto Tarklin Hill Road, and follow for a half mile to the trailhead.

To reach the Fisherman's Cove Trailhead, from Franklin, head south on Route 8 out of town. Just before it turns into a divided highway, take a right onto old Route 8. Follow it until you cross the Pecan Bridge. Then take a sharp right down a hill, and follow the sign to Seneca Hills Bible Camp. Take a right at the bottom of the hill, and follow Fisherman's Cove Road for 3 miles until you see the trailhead on your right.

Contact: Allegheny Valley Trails Association
Box 264
Franklin, PA 16323
(814) 432-4476, extension 121
www.avta-trails.org

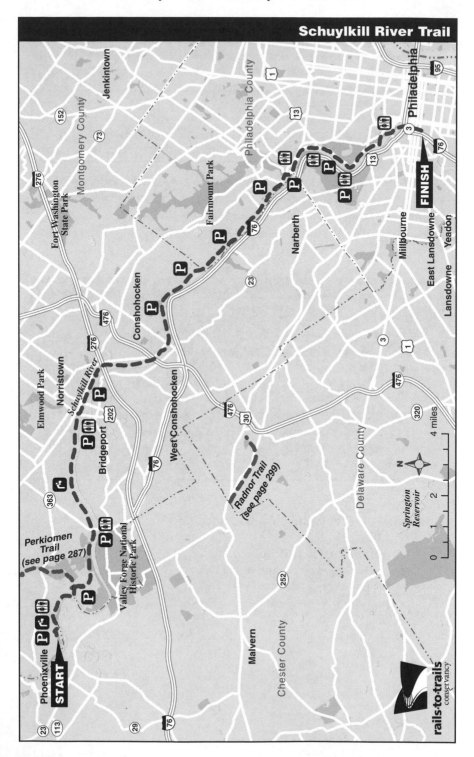

Schuylkill River Trail

Schuylkill River Trail

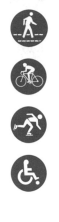

Valley Forge to Philadelphia

The Valley Forge to Philadelphia segment of the Schuylkill River Trail stretches 20.5 miles along the historic Schuylkill River from downtown Philadelphia at the Philadelphia Museum of Art out to Montgomery County and Valley Forge National Historic Park. In Philadelphia, the trail uses Fairmount Park trails and the Manayunk Canal towpath. In Montgomery County, the trail follows a former Pennsylvania Railroad line. The trail is the spine of the Schuylkill River Heritage Corridor, a five-county area designated as both a State and National Heritage Area.

Originally conceived of by the Fairmount Park Commission, the trail route grew to include many municipalities. Montgomery County constructed the trail from the Philadelphia City line to Valley Forge National Historical Park. The Chester County Department

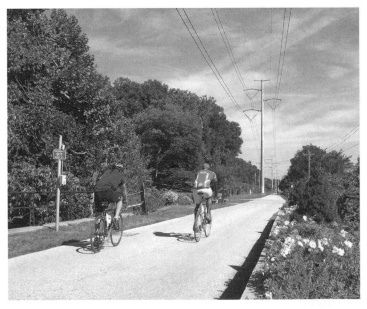

The Schuylkill River Trail is a busy commuter route during rush hour.

Location
Philadelphia, Montgomery, Berks and Schuylkill counties

Endpoints
Philadelphia to Vallley Forge

Mileage
20.5

Roughness Index
1

Surface
Asphalt

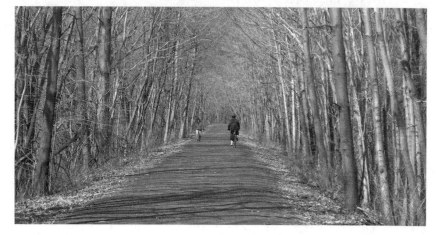

The trail is the spine of the Schuylkill River Heritage Corridor, a five-county area designated as both a state and national heritage area.

of Parks and Recreation is currently planning the section between Phoenixville and Pottstown. The Schuylkill River Greenway Association is working on the sections from the Montgomery County line to Birdsboro and from Gibraltar into Reading. And finally, the Schuylkill River Development Corporation is managing the trail construction from the Water Works in Philadelphia's Fairmount Park and along the tidal section of the Schuylkill River, known as Schuylkill Banks. The Schuylkill River Greenway Association has detailed maps of each section along with construction updates on their website.

The river was once a major transportation resource that played a key role in the region's development. Evidence of several centuries of industrial use remain where river and canal navigation, quarrying of limestone and iron ore, and production of iron and steel have succeeded each other as mainstays of the region's economy.

Today the trail is a busy commuter route during rush hour. This trail's asphalt tread is somewhat narrower than that of many of the new trails—caution, as well as rail-trail etiquette, should be heeded. This section runs parallel to the Schuylkill River, with numerous access points at businesses and public transit. In Norristown the trail connects with the 30th Street train station in downtown Philadelphia.

At Betzwood, just outside Valley Forge National Park, the trail provides a direct link to the 19.5-mile Perkiomen Trail (see page 287) and will eventually access the Cross County Trail in Conshohocken and the Chester Valley Trail in Norristown. Future development of the Schuylkill River Trail will extend it along the entire length of the Schuylkill River, more than 140 miles, from its confluence with the Delaware River to its headwaters in Schuylkill County.

Additional Schuylkill River Trail segments:

Thun Trail

The Thun Trail (pronounced *tune*) is part of the Schuylkill River Trail System. Large railroad bridges, built in 1918, provide impressive views of the Schuylkill River and the surrounding hills. Paralleling Routes 422 and 724, this section of the Schuylkill River Trail offers commuters an alternate route and leisurely riders beautiful views. It is a little more than 18 miles long. Currently a 4-mile on-road route connects the two developed segments of the trail. The western end between Reading and Gibraltar is 5.8 miles long, and the eastern developed trail segment 8.9 miles long.

John Bartram Trail

The John Bartram Trail (aka Bartram Trail) is simply one section of the very involved Schuylkill River Trail, which is being developed in sections as funds and capacity permit. Currently 9.6 miles of the Bartram Trail is open. There are three disconnected pieces of trail that have been developed for nonmotorized use. The Appalachian Trail crosses this section of the Schuylkill River Trail, southwest of the village of Port Clinton, and sections of the trail cross Pennsylvania Gamelands. You can buy fresh roasted peanuts and penny candy in Port Clinton from one of the few remaining penny candy stores in the state.

DIRECTIONS

To reach the trailhead and parking at Valley Forge National Historical Park, take the Pennsylvania Turnpike, Interstate 76, to Valley Forge, Exit 326. Take US 422 west to the Audubon/Trooper exit, and turn left off the exit ramp. You'll find parking for the Schuylkill River Trail at the Betzwood Picnic area just ahead.

To reach the Philadelphia trailhead, head west from Center City in Philadelphia on Walnut Street. Turn left on 23rd Street, right on Spruce Street, and right on South 25th Street. Before having to turn right on Locust Street, look to the left; there is a pathway to the trailhead reachable by crossing the railroad tracks at an at-grade crossing. There is no dedicated parking for this trailhead.

Contact: Schuylkill River Greenway Association
140 College Drive
Pottstown, PA 19464
(484) 945-0200
www.schuylkillriver.org

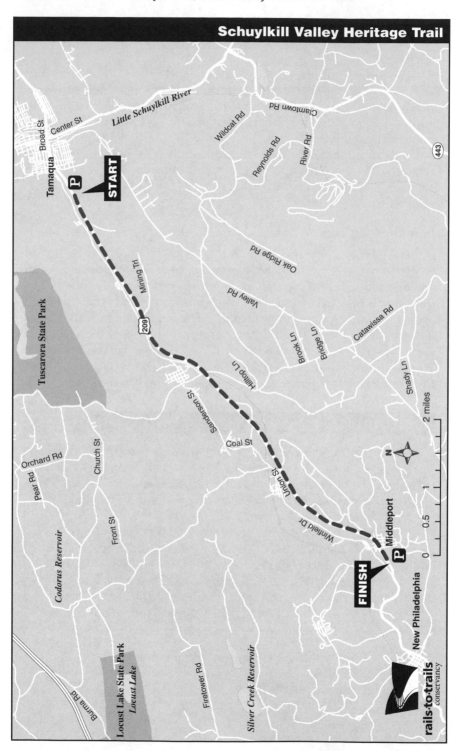

Schuylkill Valley Heritage Trail

Schuylkill Valley Heritage Trail

The Schuylkill Valley Heritage Trail passes through the rolling green hills of the Schuylkill River Valley, from just outside of Tamaqua to Middleport. The trail runs immediately adjacent to State Highway 209, and was originally intended to be part of a highway widening project. The state had already removed the old rail and ties when funding for the highway was eliminated, which then created the opportunity to build a trail.

Begin your trip at the northern end of the trail in Tamaqua, a former mining town whose historic district features many beautiful renovated structures, including the 1874 Tamaqua rail station. Officially called the Philadelphia & Reading Railroad Passenger Station, this Victorian styled station has been fully restored and is a part of the Tamaqua National Register Historic District. The station now serves as a cultural and economic center within Tamaqua.

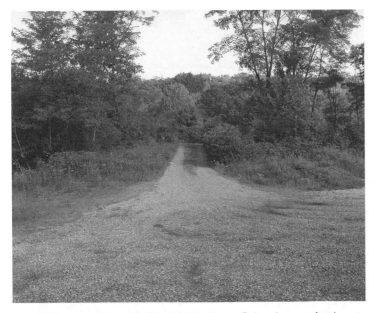

Location
Schuylkill County

Endpoints
Tamaqua to Middleport

Mileage
7.3

Roughness Index
2

Surface
Gravel and dirt

The dirt and sand base of the Schuylkill Valley Heritage Trail can become soft and unsuitable for biking in wet weather. Use caution after heavy rains.

From the parking lot you can see Newkirk Tunnel, an extinct coal mine that opened in 1868 and by the 1940s penetrated 2,211 feet into the mountainside. Now gated and leaching water from internal springs, the tunnel is part a state effort to clean water flowing from mines using a passive limestone filter that removes acid, iron and aluminum contamination. The trailhead area has signs about the mine's history and water treatment.

The route south from here to Middleport is challenging; the trail traverses undulating hills, many at maximum grade. The dirt and sand base can become soft and unsuitable for biking in wet weather. Use caution on the trail after heavy rains.

Large mile markers indicate the length of your trip, in each direction. There are plans to extend the trail to Pottsville for a total of 16 miles, but this development has not yet been scheduled.

DIRECTIONS

To reach the Tamaqua Trailhead, from Interstate 81, take Exit 131 to Highway 54 East. Continue on 54 East until the stoplight for State Route 309 in Rush. Turn right onto 309 South to Tamaqua. In Tamaqua, turn right onto State Highway 209 (West Broad Street). Continue through Tamaqua on 209. Just outside of Tamaqua, turn left at a sign for Schuylkill Valley Heritage Trail, and proceed down the short gravel road to the parking area.

To reach the Middleport Trailhead, take State Highway 209 into Middleport where it becomes Union Street. Parking is on Union Street between Washington and St. Clair streets.

Contact: Eastern Schuylkill Recreation Commission
138 West Broad Street, 3rd Floor
Tamaqua, PA 18252
(570) 668-2919
www.easternschuylkillrec.com

Snow Shoe Trail

Coordinated by the Snow Shoe Rails to Trails Association (SSRTA), the Snow Shoe Trail caters primarily to ATV and off-road motorcycle enthusiasts. It is open to other users as well, but the rough ballast and gravel surface makes for a bumpy mountain bike ride or a tricky hike.

The Snow Shoe Trail finds its origins in the Beech Creek Railroad, which opened in 1884 to serve the Clearfield Bituminous Coal Company, whose mines were expected to produce 500,000 tons for coal each year. In 1899 the railroad ceased independent operation and was incorporated into the New York Central & Hudson River Railroad Company. The rail line also offered passenger service until about 1934. The railroad saw its last train in 1990, under the ownership of the Consolidated Rail Corporation. By 1994 the tracks had been removed and the right-of-way had been acquired by the Headwaters Charitable Trust in anticipation of a rails-to-trails project. Since then the SSRTA formed and has worked to create this fully functional rail-trail.

Location
Centre and
Clearfield counties

Endpoints
Winburne to
Clarence

Mileage
18.5

Roughness Index
3

Surface
Ballast and gravel

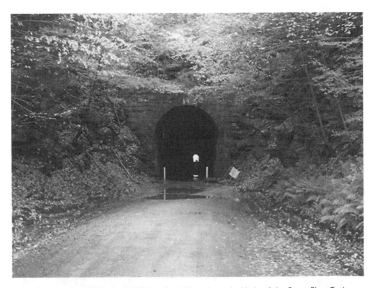

Completed in 1883, the 1,277-foot Peale Tunnel is a highlight of the Snow Shoe Trail. Bring a light to get a better look at it.

317

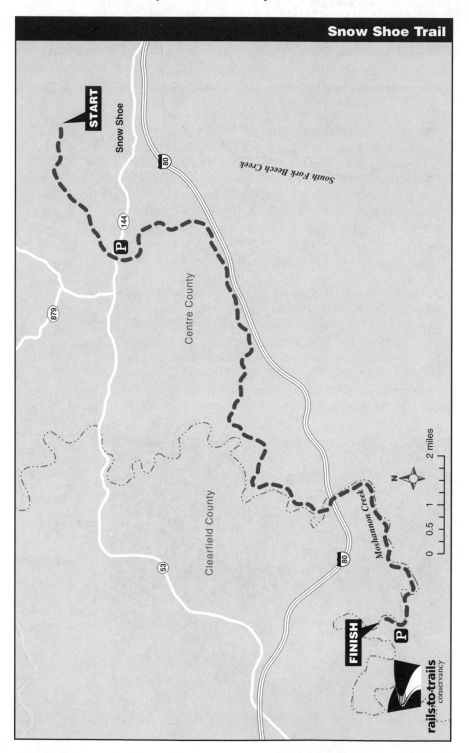

The Snow Shoe Trail preserves the 1,277-foot Peale Tunnel, completed in October 1883. If you plan to pass through the tunnel, bring a light to get a better look at the cut-stone entrances and mix of brick and natural surface on the interior. Its viaduct offers an excellent view of Moshannon Creek; though at 770 feet long and 110 feet above the creek, the bridge may be unnerving for those with a fear of heights.

While all types of users are welcome on the trail, motorized users *must* get a permit from SSRTA. Local ATV membership is highly recommended. Obey all of the posted signs and be courteous to other trail users.

DIRECTIONS

To reach the Gillentown Trailhead, take Interstate 80 to Exit 147 for Snow Shoe. Turn left and head north on Route 144. Continue approximately 3.5 miles. You will pass Seperish Recycling on the left. At the bottom of the hill beyond the recycling center, turn left at the Snow Shoe Trail trailhead sign. Continue down the gravel road to the large gravel parking lot. The trail is clearly visible along the length of the parking area.

Contact: Snow Shoe Rails to Trails Association
P.O. Box 314
Clarence, PA 16829
www.ssrt.org

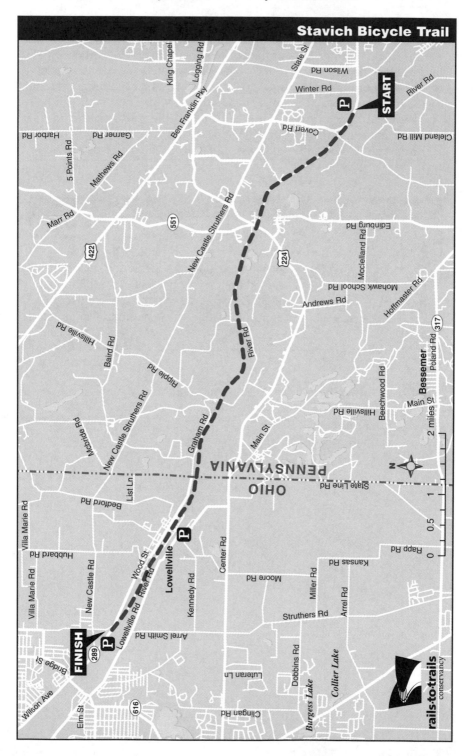

Stavich Bicycle Trail

Stavich Bicycle Trail

onstructed in 1983 with the help of donations from the Stavich family and local individuals, the Stavich Trail is unusual in several ways. First, unlike most rail-trails, it was built on an interurban electric railroad right-of-way—the Penn-Ohio trolley line, which fell into disuse in 1933. Because interurban railroads were not built to the stringent standards of conventional railroads, you'll encounter more hills than you might on other rail-trails.

The Stavich's second notable feature is the fact that it is among the growing number of rail-trails in the country that connects two states. This gently rolling trail takes you from near New Castle, Pennsylvania, to Struthers, Ohio. Running along the Mahoning River, this mostly rural, paved trail is great for bicycling, inline skating, walking and is accessible for persons with disabilities.

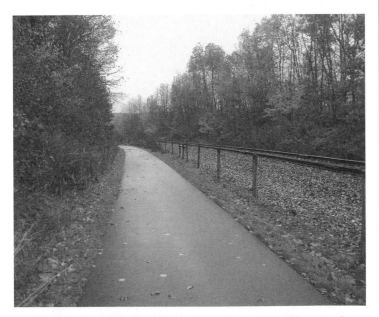

The Stavich Bicycle Trail is among the growing number of rail-trails in the country that connects two states.

Location
Lawrence County

Endpoints
New Castle,
Pennsylvania, to
Struthers, Ohio

Mileage
10

**Roughness
Index**
1

Surface
Asphalt

Lastly, this is a rail-with-trail that shares the right-of-way with an active CSX rail line for part of the trail's route. Recent detailed research from RTC suggests rail-with-trails, which are growing in popularity around the country, offer communities both safe and enjoyable recreation and transportation options. The U.S. Department of the Interior named the Stavich Bicycle Trail a National Recreation Trail in 2003.

DIRECTIONS

To reach the Pennsylvania Trailhead, take State Route 60 to State Street (Highway 224 East). Continue to Scotland Lane. Turn right and right again onto Washington Street. Washington Street leads to the well-marked trailhead.

To get to the western trailhead in Ohio, take State Highway 224 west to Poland, Ohio. Turn right onto State Route 616, and follow it across the Mahoning River. Just after the river, turn right onto Broad Street. The trailhead is on the right in about a mile.

This trail is wheelchair-accessible.

Contact: Ohio Bikeways
www.ohiobikeways.net/stavich.htm

Stony Valley Railroad Grade

O riginally named St. Anthony's Wilderness by Moravian missionaries who arrived in the colony in 1742 to convert Native tribes, the Stony Creek Valley became the site of five bustling towns after discovery of coal in 1824. The Schuylkill & Susquehanna Railroad was built in the 1850s to transport coal to the canals and tourists to enjoy the healing mineral waters at Cold Springs. The spring water's popularity led to the construction of a 200-room resort to accommodate the wealthy Philadelphians who came for the healing waters.

By 1944, the mines were exhausted, the lumber stripped, and the railroad fell into disuse. The elegant, 200-room resort hotel at Cold Springs burned to the

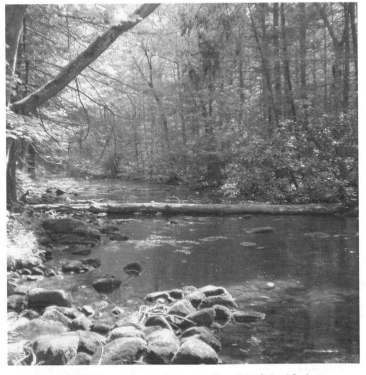

Located on 44,342 acres of state game land, the Stony Valley Railroad Grade passes through natural habitat with an abundance of wildlife.

Location
Dauphin, Lebanon and Schuylkill counties

Endpoints
Stony Valley Road in Ellendale to Lebanon Valley Reservoir in Pine Grove Township

Mileage
21

Roughness Index
3

Surface
Dirt and gravel

323

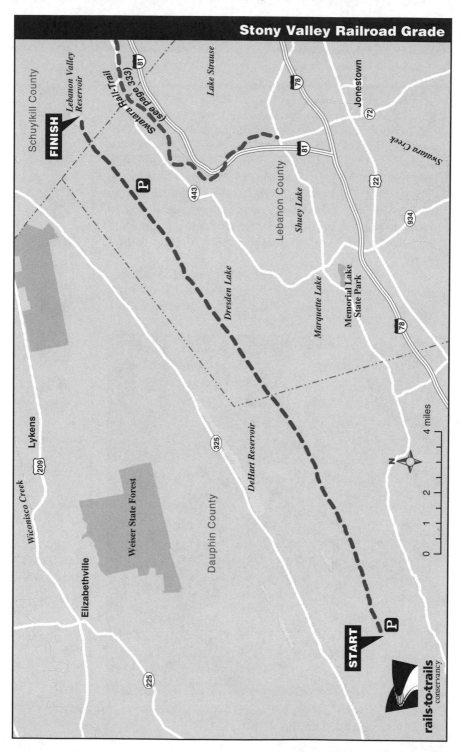

Stony Valley Railroad Grade

ground. The Pennsylvania Game Commission purchased the land in 1945 and converted the railroad corridor to a trail soon after, making the Stony Valley Railroad Grade one of the nation's earliest rail-trails.

Located on 44,342 acres of state game land, the trail passes through natural habitat with an abundance of wildlife. Little evidence of the once thriving town of Cold Springs remains. The foundation and stone steps to the old Cold Springs Hotel are now hidden beneath towering Norway spruces planted by the hotel's original landscapers.

Unique among rail-trails in Pennsylvania, each fall the Stony Valley Railroad Grade is open to motor vehicles for one day. During hunting season, the trail is closed to non-hunting bicycle and equestrian use. Hunters with the appropriate license and weapon can bicycle to their quarry. Located a few miles north of Harrisburg, the state capital, the trail can be a busy place in the fall and during hunting season. As with all rail-trails located along state game lands, check with the game commission for trail status prior to your visit.

DIRECTIONS

To reach the western trailhead, at Ellendale, from Harrisburg, take Route 322 north, exiting at Dauphin. Turn right at the stop sign and right again at the T at the end of the street. Turn left onto Stony Creek Road and continue for 5 miles to Ellendale. You will see a dirt road off to the right, which looks like a cul-de-sac but continues. Follow the dirt road to the gated trailhead and parking lot.

To reach the eastern trailhead, from the Harrisburg area, take Interstate 81 north to Exit 90. At the end of the ramp, turn left onto Lickdale Road. Immediately turn left again onto State Route 1001 (becomes Gold Mine Road), and follow it for 7.2 miles. At the top of the mountain, turn left onto Old Railroad Bed Road. The trailhead and parking are straight ahead.

Contact: Pennsylvania Game Commission
2001 Elmerton Avenue
Harrisburg, PA 17110
(717) 787-9612
www.pgc.state.pa.us/portal/server.pt/community/pgc/9106

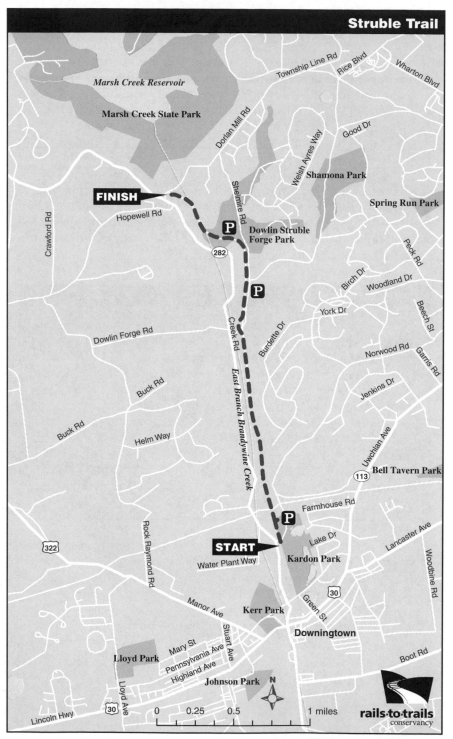

Struble Trail

Struble Trail

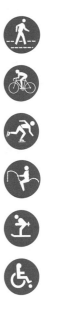

The Chester County Parks & Recreation Department opened this trail in 1979 on part of a former Pennsylvania Railroad right-of-way. Today the 2.6-mile trail attracts more than 125,000 visitors each year.

Named for the late Robert G. Struble, a teacher, conservationist, county commissioner and Brandywine Valley Association executive director, the pretty trail parallels the East Branch of Brandywine Creek for a short distance. The trail's flat surface makes a perfect setting for amateur naturalists and a tranquil venue for joggers, bicyclists, inline skaters and cross-country skiers. Equestrians are welcome on the undeveloped sections of the trail.

The trail begins right near the downtown section of the pleasant borough of Downingtown right off Norwood Road. Traveling north, the trail cuts through pleasant wooded areas, a pristine setting in this rural

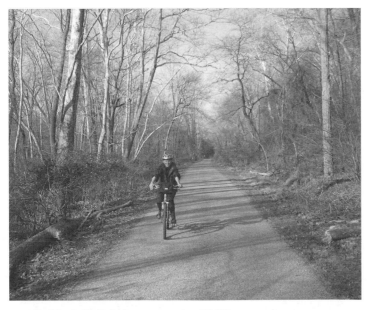

The 2.6-mile Struble Trail attracts more than 125,000 visitors each year.

Location
Chester County

Endpoints
Downingtown
to Dorlan

Mileage
2.6

**Roughness
Index**
1

Surface
Asphalt

327

section of southeastern Pennsylvania. You cross only one road during this journey—Dowlin Forge Road, which doesn't see much traffic. Currently, the trail connects to the 2-mile Uwchlan Trail on the right just beyond this road crossing, which links to residential and commercial sections throughout the township. Currently the trail ends south of Marsh Creek Park in Dorlan; however, there are loose plans to develop it farther to the north.

DIRECTIONS

To reach the Norwood Road Trailhead, from US Highway 30 Bypass traveling west, exit at Route 282 near Downingtown. Turn left off the exit and proceed on Norwood Road under the US Highway 30 bridge. Turn at the second drive on the right, where you see the trailhead.

To reach the Norwood Road Trailhead, from US Highway 30 Bypass traveling east, exit at US 322. Turn right and go to Pennsylvania Avenue in Downingtown. Turn left on Pennsylvania Avenue and proceed to State Route 282. Turn left on State Route 282. Follow and turn right onto Norwood Road. The trailhead is the first left. There is a sign for the parking lot.

This trail is wheelchair-accessible.

Contact: Chester County Parks and Recreation
601 Westtown Road, Suite 160
West Chester, PA 19380
(610) 344-6415
www.chesco.org/ccparks

Susquehanna Warrior Trail

This Susquehanna Warrior Trail is nestled in the beautiful Susquehanna River Valley, lush with green meadows and surrounding mountain peaks. Eventually the trail will cover 18.5 miles, but now it totals about 10 miles in loosely connected sections. Most of the trail currently runs from north of Berwick to Hunlock between Route 11 and the Susquehanna River on the corridor of the old Delaware, Lehigh and Western railroad beds.

Start at the southern endpoint north of Berwick at the Pennsylvania Power and Light (PPL) Riverlands Park. A nice destination unto itself, the park has picnic tables, playgrounds, a small lake for fishing and a crushed stone loop path to enjoy.

From the parking lot, the trail heads north and runs adjacent to the active railroad tracks with a slight grade separation. You pass through quiet, pretty woods for approximately 1.5 miles before the trail abruptly ends at

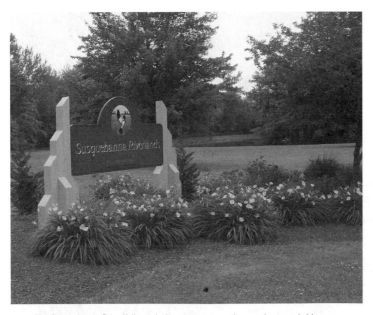

The Susquehanna River Valley is lush with green meadows and surrounded by mountain peaks.

Location
Columbia and Luzerne counties

Endpoints
Pennsylvania Power and Light Riverlands Park to Hunlock Creek Garden Drive-In Theater

Mileage
10

Roughness Index
1

Surface
Crushed stone

329

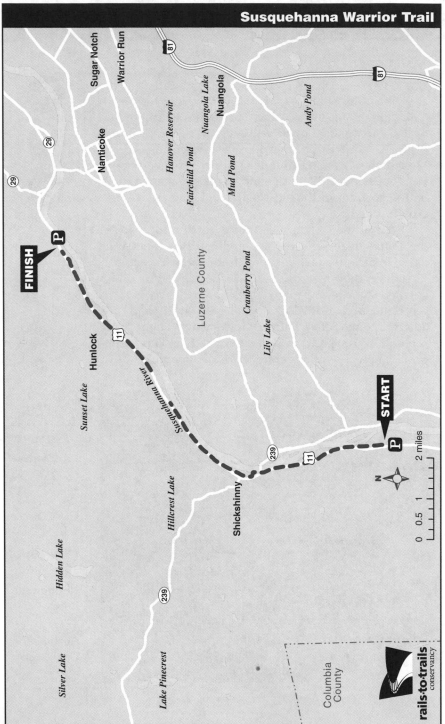

Susquehanna Warrior Trail

81

81

Sugar Notch

Warrior Run

Nanticoke

29

29

Hanover Reservoir

Fairchild Pond

Nuangola Lake

Nuangola

Mud Pond

Andy Pond

Luzerne County

Cranberry Pond

Lily Lake

FINISH

P

11

Hunlock

Sunset Lake

Susquehanna River

START

P

11

239

Shickshinny

Hillcrest Lake

N

2 miles

0   0.5   1

Hidden Lake

239

Lake Pinecrest

Silver Lake

Columbia County

rails-to-trails
conservancy

the entrance to a privately owned junkyard. You can't miss this endpoint—the trail is blocked by two junkyard cars. Bear left and head out to Route 11 for a brief quarter-mile ride to the parking lot entrance of the junkyard. From here the trail continues north alongside Route 11.

As you approach Shickshinny, the trail ends at the bridge crossing. Shickshinny is the best spot along the route to stop for something to eat. To pick up the trail again, follow Route 11, pass the bridge and go approximately one-eighth of a mile before turning right onto East Butler Street. Follow it a short distance down to South Susquehanna Street, where the trail resumes.

You'll find yourself closer to the river again for a 3-mile stretch. The trail gradually gets closer to Route 11 as it travels north, eventually stopping at a guardrail on Route 11.

Travel north on Route 11 approximately 1 mile to find the next trail segment at a firing range. Portions of this final segment are right next to Route 11, but other sections veer off closer to the river and into green space where you see another pretty bridge as well as another junkyard. The trail ends at the Garden Drive-In, one of the country's few remaining drive-in movie theaters. If you time your visit right, take in a show at the end of your ride or walk.

DIRECTIONS

To reach the southern trailhead north of Berwick, take 239 North into Shickshinny and turn left onto State Route 11 South. Follow State Route 11 South approximately 3.5 miles to the Pennsylvania Power and Light Riverlands Park entrance on the left. Ample parking is available.

To reach the northern trailhead in Hunlock Creek, take 239 North into Shickshinny and turn right onto State Route 11 North. Follow State Route 11 North approximately 8 miles to the Garden Drive-In. Turn right at the drive-in. Look for signs for the trail and a trail parking lot on your immediate right.

This trail is wheelchair-accessible.

Contact: Susquehanna Warrior Trail Council
P.O. Box 54
Shickshinny, PA 18655
(570) 696-5082
www.susquehannawarriortrail.org

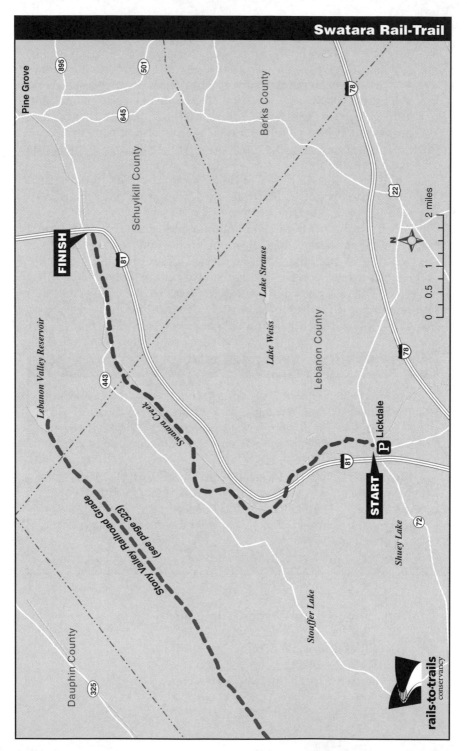

Swatara Rail-Trail

Swatara Rail-Trail

The discovery of anthracite coal in the Tremont area of Pennsylvania shaped commerce and development well into the 1800s. The Union Canal was constructed in the 1820s to connect the Schuylkill and Susquehanna rivers and improve transport of anthracite coal. A branch canal was constructed from Lebanon to Pine Grove through what is now Swatara State Park. The Flood of 1862 destroyed the branch. By then because the Lebanon-Tremont Branch of the Reading Railroad on the opposite bank of Swatara Creek served all transport needs, the canal was never repaired.

The Swatara Rail-Trail stretches 10 miles along Swatara Creek from Pine Grove almost to Lickdale, revealing remnants of both the canal and the railroad along the way. Even though the path is somewhat close to Interstate 81, the lush forest surroundings and rugged trail surface create a sense of remoteness perfect for the adventure lover.

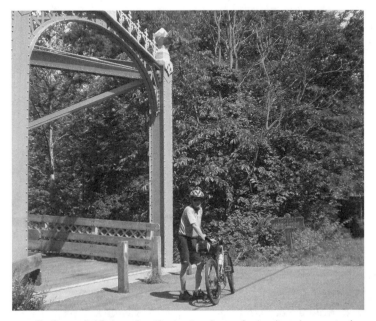

The Swatara Rail-Trail stretches 10 miles along Swatara Creek and reveals remnants of both the canal and the railroad along the way.

Location
Lebanon and
Schuylkill counties

Endpoints
Exit 90, Interstate
81, in Lickdale to
Exit 100, Interstate
81 in Pine Grove

Mileage
10

**Roughness
Index**
3

Surface
Gravel

333

Swatara State Park covers more than 3,500 acres of land but has no formal entrance or recreation center. The park's main activities are paddling and fishing in the Swatara Creek that flows through it. The woodlands surrounding the creek and rail-trail provide good cover for deer and fowl in this hunting area popular among the local population. Although the trail starts and ends outside the park's boundaries, the majority is within it.

Some islands in the creek have primitive campsites, but the park remains undeveloped. It doesn't have signs or facilities. The park's office is located at Memorial Lake State Park about 10 miles south on Interstate 81. Trail maintenance is limited to mowing and drainage infill with large stones. Volunteers have placed wood mileage markers along the trail, but there is no other signage.

At one section the trail is an unused paved road. Nearby, a few miles north, the Stony Valley Railroad Grade (see page 323) offers another backcountry treat; an extended day or weekend excursion on both trails may be in order. The trail also connects to the Appalachian Trail near Inwood.

The Swatara Trail ends in unmowed grass behind the Hampton Inn along I-81, with several food services nearby.

DIRECTIONS

To reach the Lickdale Campground trailhead, travel north on Interstate 81 from Harrisburg about 20 miles to Exit 90. Follow the signs for Lebanon. At the first stoplight, continue straight, then immediately turn left into the private campground parking lot. Parking and trailhead access are to the right of and behind the camp store. The trail leads out of the parking area to the north and is heavy ballast for the first 100 yards because the campground vehicular traffic uses it. The only parking for this trail is at private Lickdale Campground off I-81.

There is no formal access at the northeast endpoint, but the trail can be accessed at the grassy area below the Hampton Inn parking lot off Exit 100 of Interstate 81.

Contact: Memorial Lake and Swatara State Parks
RR 1, Box 704
Grantville, PA 17028
(717) 865-6470
www.dcnr.state.pa.us/stateparks/parks/swatara.aspx

Switchback Railroad Trail

When it began operating, the Switchback Railroad was the second railroad in America and the first in Pennsylvania. Built to haul coal from the Summit Mine to the Lehigh Canal, the railroad evolved from a gravity-powered system (The Down Track) and mule-powered system (The Back Track) to a 95 percent gravity-run operation.

In the late 1800s as steam locomotion became more commonplace, the Switchback Railroad was needed less for coal transport but was adapted into a passenger operation. From 1870 and for the next six decades, the Switchback Gravity Railroad evolved into a popular tourist attraction—one that thrilled visitors with 50 mile-per-hour rides downhill through the lush landscape of the Lehigh Valley. It is credited with inspiring the creation of the roller coaster. The tourist attraction closed in 1929, and the Switchback was sold for scrap in 1937 and converted to a trail in 1977.

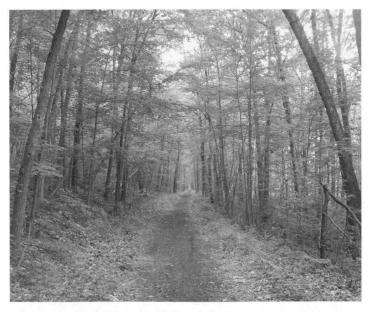

With its hard-packed dirt surface, the Down Track is the easier southern route.

Location
Carbon County

Endpoints
Summit Hill to
Jim Thorpe

Mileage
18

**Roughness
Index**
3

Surface
Dirt, gravel and
ballast

335

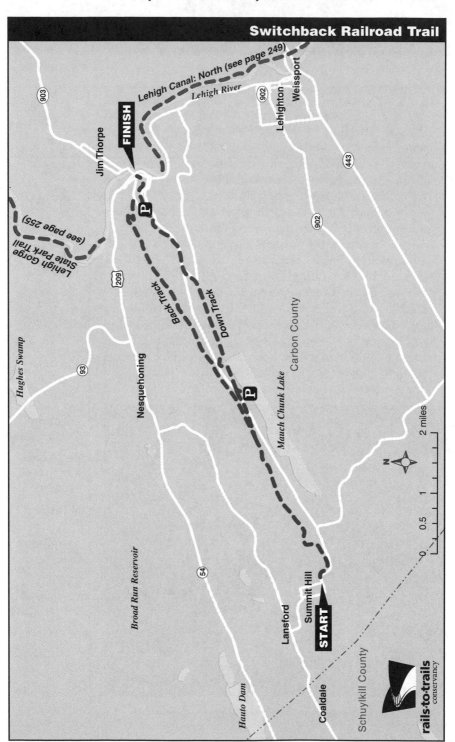

Today, the Switchback Trail still inspires tourists and locals alike. Two 9-mile routes intersect to make up the Switchback. Regardless of which you choose, start in Summit Hill and bike downhill toward Jim Thorpe. The grade in reverse is challenging. Although this trail doesn't require a lot of pedaling, it commands your attention. (For a shorter ride, pick up the trail in Mauch Chunk Lake Park, which has parking, restrooms, picnic areas and campgrounds. Fishing is permitted.)

With its hard-packed dirt surface, the Down Track is the easier southern route. This track takes you along Mauch Chunk Lake for a half mile and then plunges into a lush forested area. At mile 7, the trail ends abruptly on Lentz Trail Road. Cross the road, head downhill toward Jim Thorpe, and continue past the power plant entrance (go around the gated drive), and pick up the trail again at the back of the power plant access road. From here continue on a peaceful wooded trail, riding on a bluff overlooking the community of Jim Thorpe below.

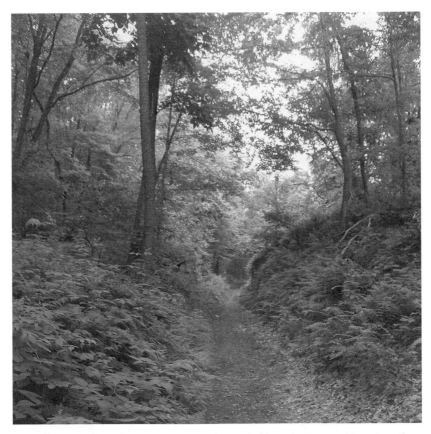

Pay attention as you traverse ballast, navigate large rocks in packed dirt, and portage your bike on the northern Back Track.

The northern Back Track is recommended only for mountain bikes. Be prepared to pay attention as you traverse ballast, navigate large rocks in packed dirt, and portage your bike around sections of the trail that are too steep to cross otherwise. As this section of the trail winds down outside Jim Thorpe you'll discover an optional small loop that takes you to a scenic overview. Beware: Locals say copperheads have been seen in that area. At the trail's end, you will encounter a knee-breaking descent on a steep, slippery rock surface where keeping your footing while holding your bike will be challenging.

Bike rental and shuttle services available in downtown Jim Thorpe will drop you off at the trailhead in Summit Hill, where you can take the Switchback Trail downhill right back into town and spend the rest of your day enjoying the many quaint shops and restaurants. If you'd rather keep exploring trails, the area has several other rail-trails to explore including the Lehigh Canal: North (or D&L Trail, see page 249) and the Lehigh Gorge State Park Trail (see page 255).

DIRECTIONS

To reach the Summit Hill Trailhead, take Interstate 476 to Exit 74, then take US Highway 209 South to Jim Thorpe. In Jim Thorpe, turn left onto Broadway, which becomes Lentz Trail Road. Continue past the Mauch Chunk Lake Park entrance. At the intersection of State Route 902 turn right. Travel 2 miles until 902 turns sharply right in Summit Hill. Take that right and make another, immediate right on Holland Street. The trailhead is at the end of this street. There is no official parking at this trailhead.

To reach the Down Track Trailhead in Jim Thorpe, take Interstate 476 to Exit 74, then take 209 South to Jim Thorpe. Follow 209 past the train station, and turn left onto Center Street. Take a right on Pine Avenue and left on North Street. There is a trailhead one-eighth of a mile up on your right. (This rocky steep ascent is not recommended as a start point.)

The trail can also be easily accessed from its midpoint at Mauch Chunk Lake Park, outside Jim Thorpe off Lentz Trail Road.

Contact: Mauch Chunk Lake Park Office
Caron County Parks & Recreation
625 Lentz Trail Road
Jim Thorpe, PA 18229
(570) 329-3669
http://switchbackgravityrr.org/sbtrail.htm

Warren to North Warren Bike Trail

L ocated along the banks of Conewango Creek, the open 3-mile segment of this proposed 11-mile trail follows an old New York Central branch north from the city of Warren. Designed to serve primarily as a safe, off-road route for cyclists and commuters, from the downtown area to the burgeoning North Warren business district along Route 62, the trail also preserves scenic vistas of the Conewango and controls flooding along its tributary, Jackson Run.

Northwestern Pennsylvania history is defined by early oil exploration and the industry and community development it brought to the area. Warren is a classic example of a community that saw large growth when oil was first discovered. The New York Central railroad corridor this trail follows was built to serve the several oil refineries that once occupied this area.

Beginning at the north end of East Street in downtown Warren, the trail leads north out of town, following the banks of quiet Conewango Creek. It is not uncommon to see wildlife near the river's edge, including ducks, deer and abundant bird life.

Location
Warren County

Endpoints
Warren to
North Warren

Mileage
3

**Roughness
Index**
1

Surface
Asphalt

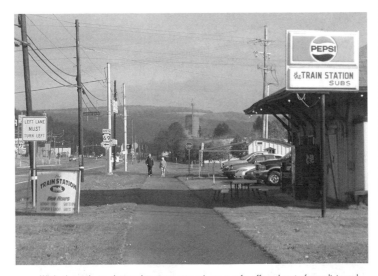

While the trail was designed to serve primarily as a safe, off-road route for cyclists and commuters, it also preserves the scenic vistas of the Conewango.

339

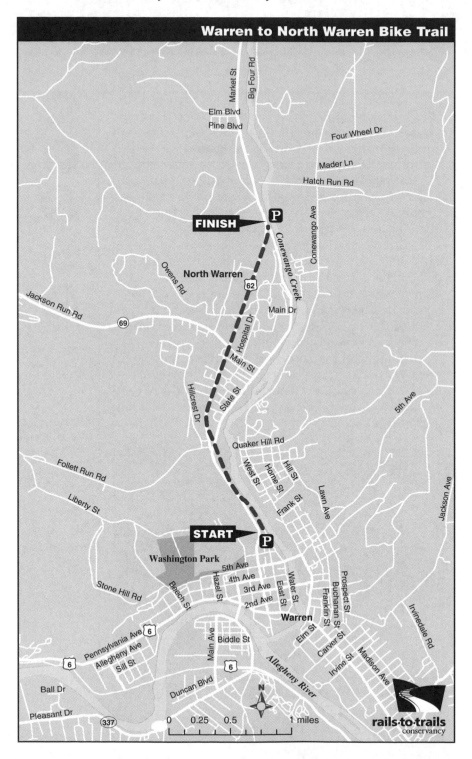

As the trail continues north, it leaves the creek and enters a busy commercial section along Route 62. The trail is sufficiently removed from the highway, creating a pleasant buffer from traffic. There are a number of restaurants and shops along this section to North Warren. The trail ends near a beautiful town park that has picnic areas, a garden, parking and restrooms.

DIRECTIONS

To reach the East Street Trailhead, exit US Highway 6 for Ludlow Street, follow it north and take a right onto Business Route 6. Follow Business Route 6 (Pennsylvania Avenue) to Market Street (Route 62). Turn left on Market Street and continue to 5th Avenue. Turn right on 5th Avenue and turn left on East Street. Continue to the end of the road, which has parking and the trailhead.

To reach the North Warren Trailhead, exit US Highway 6 for Ludlow Street, follow it north and take a right onto Business Route 6. Follow Business Route 6 (Pennsylvania Avenue) to Market Street (Route 62). Turn left on Market Street. Continue north until you reach North State Street in North Warren. You will see parking and the trailhead on your right.

This trail is wheelchair-accessible.

Contact: Warren County Planning & Zoning Commission
207 West 5th Avenue
Warren, PA 16365
(814) 726-386
www.warrencountypa.net

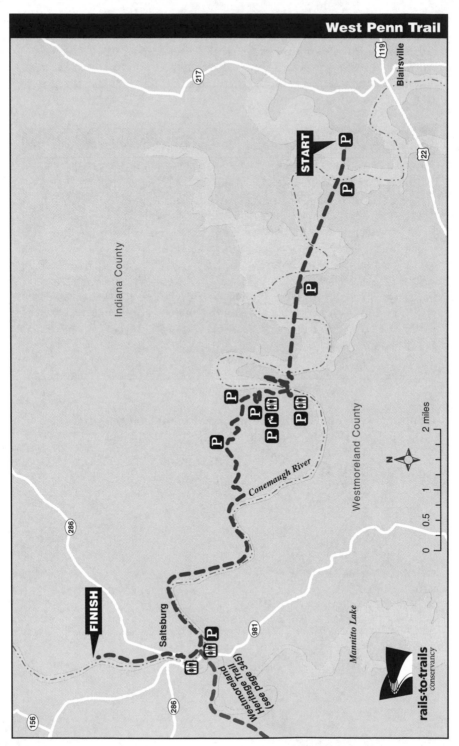

West Penn Trail

T he West Penn Trail runs largely along the corridor of the Portage Railroad line that operated from 1830 to 1864 between Pittsburgh and Harrisburg. Since the first trail section opened, the West Penn Trail has been extended to cover more than 12 miles. It is made up of five sections: 1) Conemaugh River Lake Section, near the Conemaugh Dam, passes over four stone arch bridges dating back to the early 1900s. 2) Bow Ridge Switchback to Conemaugh Dam Section passes two tunnels and a hydroelectric plant. This challenging

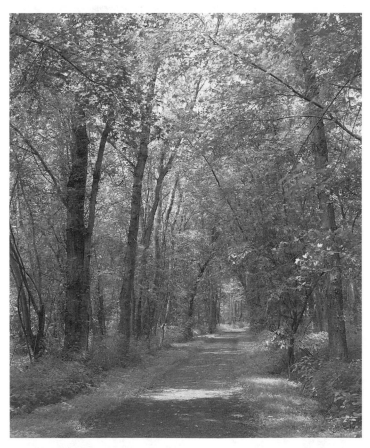

Location
Indiana and
Westmoreland
counties

Endpoints
Blairsville to
Saltsburg

Mileage
12

**Roughness
Index**
2

Surface
Crushed limestone,
dirt and asphalt

The Saltsburg Section of the trail hugs the banks of the Conemaugh River for more than 4 miles, passing through beautiful woodlands filled with lush green vegetation during warmer months.

343

section is great for extreme bikers. 3) The Dick Mayer Section follows a former railroad bed and is challenging as well. 4) The Saltsburg Section hugs the banks of the Conemaugh River for more than 4 miles, passing through beautiful woodlands filled with lush green vegetation during warmer months. Horseback riding is permitted here. 5) The Kiski Extension Section continues along the east riverbank for a mile and half where it comes to an open field. Past this point the trail becomes private property and has two washouts that are not passable by bicycle.

Two main events are held in Saltsburg each year: an annual Native American Festival and a three-day Canal Day Festival with live music, crafts, food, games and fireworks. The West Penn Trail is steadily being extended. Before you visit, check the Conemaugh Valley Conservancy website for current route information.

DIRECTIONS

To reach the Saltsburg Trailhead, from downtown Pittsburgh, take Interstate 376 (Parkway East) 12 miles to Monroeville, where Interstate 376 becomes US Route 22. Follow US Route 22 for about 18 miles to State Route 981 North at New Alexandria. Turn left on PA 981 North and continue about 8 miles to State Route 286 to State Route 981 toward Saltsburg. Cross the bridge over the Kiskiminetas River into Saltsburg. Turn on Salts Street and go three blocks. The trailhead parking will be on your right near the playground.

Contact: Conemaugh Valley Conservancy
P.O. Box 502
Hollsopple, PA 15935
(814) 479-7162
www.conemaughvalleyconservancy.org

Westmoreland Heritage Trail

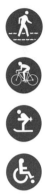

The recently opened Westmoreland Heritage Trail is an excellent example of a family-friendly multi-use rail-trail. This crushed-limestone trail features reclaimed railroad bridges over the Conemaugh River and Loyalhanna Creek, both offering great views of the river hydraulics below. The trail offers opportunities for bird watchers and other naturalists as well.

The Westmoreland Heritage Trail runs along a section of the former Penn Central rail line, which fell into disuse in 1972. The rail line was originally opened in 1852 by a subsidiary of the Pennsylvania Railroad Company, led by George Westinghouse, Jr., to connect Saltsburg and Export. The line served to transport both passengers and freight between the many towns along its route.

Even on the hottest summer day, as you will find yourself enveloped in a lush deciduous canopy, on this scenic trail. A portion of it runs along a small tributary

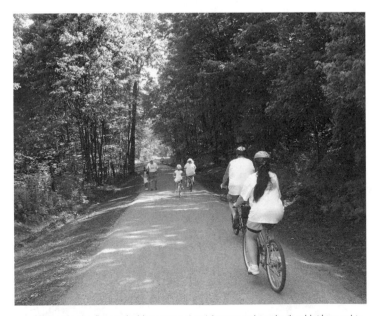

This multi-use, flat, crushed limestone rail-trail features reclaimed railroad bridges and is family friendly.

Location
Westmoreland County

Endpoints
Saltsburg to Slickville

Mileage
5

Roughness Index
1

Surface
Crushed stone

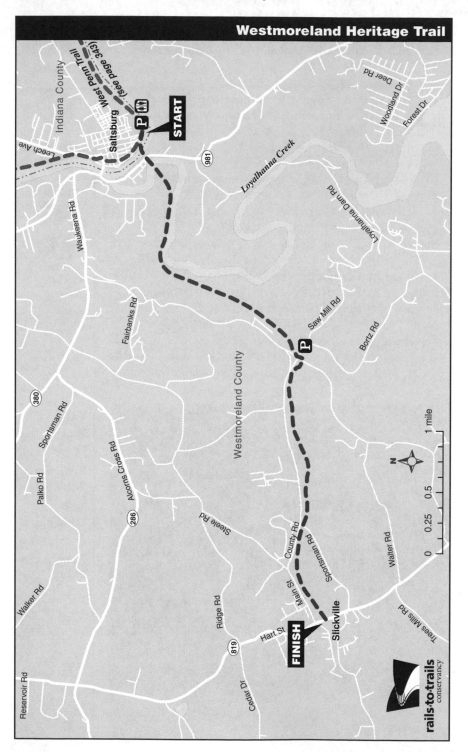

that attracts various wildlife, and natural seeps can been seen in the limestone railroad cuts at various points. At its eastern end, in Saltsburg the Westmoreland Heritage Trail connects to the West Penn Trail (see page 343). The Westmoreland Trail has a distinct uphill grade virtually the entire 5-mile length from Saltsburg to Slickville, offering a fine opportunity for a quick downhill ride back to Saltsburg.

DIRECTIONS

To reach the Saltsburg Trailhead, from Blairsville, take Highway 22 West. Turn right onto 981 North, toward Saltsburg. In approximately 7.5 miles, turn right onto Washington Street, and take the bridge across the river into Saltsburg. Go 500 feet and turn right onto Salt Street. The street bears left and becomes Canal Street. At the end of Canal Street, turn right into the small public playground parking area near the playground equipment. Both the Westmoreland Heritage Trail and the West Penn Trail can be accessed here. This trail is wheelchair-accessible.

Contact: Regional Trail Corporation
Westmoreland Heritage Trail Chapter
RR #12, Box 203
Greensburg, PA 15601
(724) 872-5586
www.co.westmoreland.pa.us/parks/cwp/view.
asp?a=3&q=619986

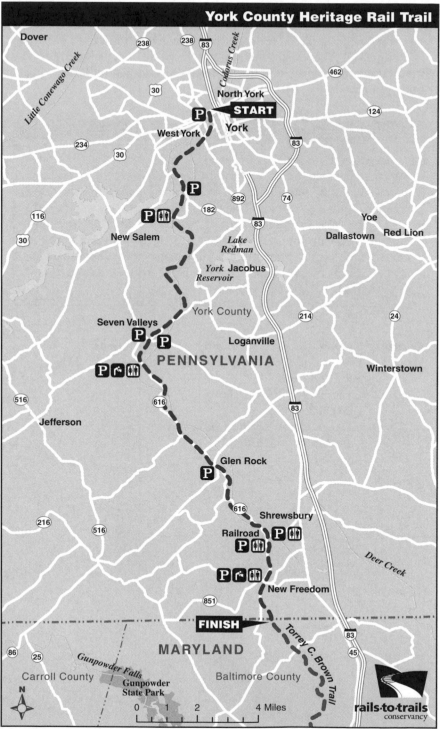

York County Heritage Rail Trail

Dover

238   238   83   *Cohorus Creek*

462

30

North York

P   **START**

West York   York   124

234

30   892   74   83

116   182

Yoe

New Salem   Dallastown   Red Lion

Lake Redman

York Jacobus
Reservoir

York County

Seven Valleys   214   24

Loganville

PENNSYLVANIA

516   616   Winterstown

Jefferson   83

Glen Rock

216   516   616   Shrewsbury

Railroad

New Freedom

851

FINISH

Deer Creek

86   25   MARYLAND   83   45

Gunpowder Falls

Carroll County   Baltimore County

Gunpowder
State Park

N

0   1   2   4 Miles

Torrey C. Brown Trail

rails·to·trails
conservancy

York County Heritage Rail Trail

T he York County Heritage Rail Trail (also called the Heritage Rail Trail County Park) winds for 21 miles through urban and rural landscapes between the City of York and the Maryland state line. The trail starts in York behind a replication of the town's colonial courthouse. Heading south, the trail passes through an urban landscape along the banks of Codorus Creek.

After a little more than a mile the trail leaves the city and enters rural countryside where the trail is flanked by fields and forests. About a mile and a half south of the Brillhart Station Trailhead is the 370-foot-long Howard Tunnel. At milepost 11 the borough of Seven Valleys provides an opportunity for refreshments at the cafe, tavern or wine shop.

A half mile farther south is the restored Hanover Junction train station. The station has been restored to appear as it did in 1863. The next 4 miles of the trail runs through farmlands and along the banks of Codorus Creek. The trail passes through Glen Rock, Railroad and

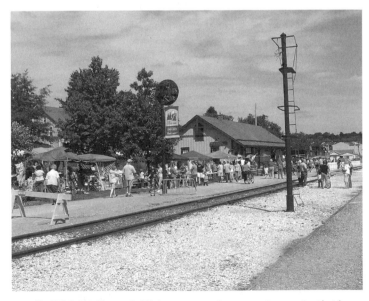

The York County Heritage Rail Trail enjoys tremendous community support, evident from events like this festival.

Location
York County

Endpoints
West Philadelphia Street and North Pershing Avenue in York to the Maryland state line

Mileage
21

Roughness Index
2

Surface
Crushed stone

New Freedom over the next 9 miles, each town providing opportunities to explore the area's rich history. From New Freedom's restored railroad station it is just a mile and a half to the Mason-Dixon Line and the connection to Maryland's 20-mile Torrey C. Brown Trail.

DIRECTIONS

To reach the York Trailhead, from Interstate 83 take Exit 22 (North George Street). Follow North George Street south for approximately 3 miles. Turn right to West Philadelphia Street. Go two blocks and turn right onto Pershing Avenue. Parking for trail users is on the west side of the street.

To reach the New Freedom Trailhead, from Interstate 83 take Exit 4 (Shrewsbury). Go west on PA Route 851. Turn left onto Main Street. At the next traffic light, Constitution Avenue, turn right. Turn right onto Franklin Street. Turn right onto Front Street. Parking is on the north side of the train station.

Contact: York County Parks
400 Mundis Race Road
York, PA 17402
(717) 840-7440
www.yorkcountyparks.org/parkpages/railtrail.htm

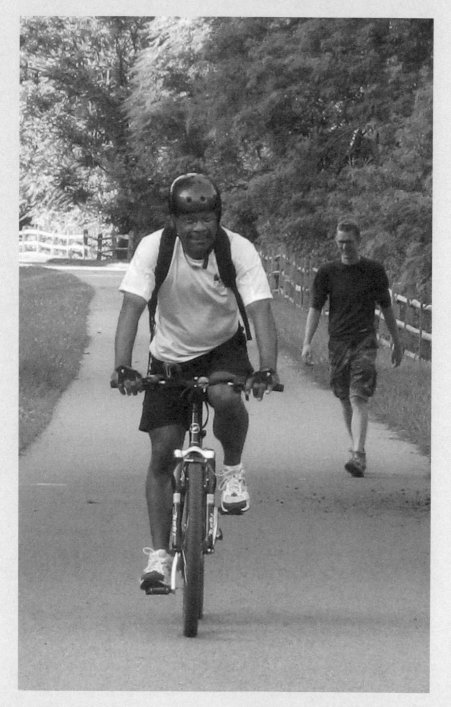

The 16-mile Butler-Freeport Community Trail traces a wooded valley about an hour and a half north of Pittsburgh.

STAFF PICKS

Best Rail-Trails

When Rails-to-Trails Conservancy staff members scoured the Northeast for the best rail-trails, these were the ones that stood out as the best. Short or long, city or country, these are rail-trails not to miss.

New Jersey
Atlantic County Bikeway
Columbia Trail
Paulinskill Valley Trail

New York
Allegheny River Valley Trail
Genesee Valley Greenway
Harlem Valley Rail Trail
Heritage Trail
High Line
Lehigh Valley Trail Linear
 Park—Victor to Rush
Mohawk-Hudson Bike-Hike Trail
Ontario Pathways Rail Trail
Walk Over the Hudson
Wallkill Valley Rail Trail

Pennsylvania
Allegheny River Trail
Clarion–Little Toby Creek Trail
Ghost Town Trail
Great Allegheny Passage
Ironton Rail-Trail
Lebanon Valley Rail-Trail
Lehigh Canal
Lehigh Gorge State Park Trail
Oil Creek State Park Trail
Perkiomen Trail
Pine Creek Trail
Roaring Run
Schuylkill River Trail
Stavich Bicycle Trail
Stony Valley Railroad Grade
West Penn Trail
York County Heritage Rail Trail

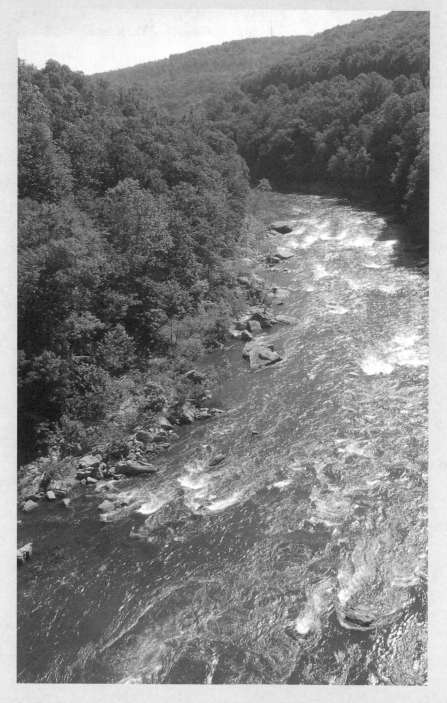

The Great Allegheny Passage showcases the Youghiogheny River, a popular whitewater rafting destination.

ACKNOWLEDGMENTS

Each of the trails in *Rail-Trails Pennsylvania, New Jersey and New York* was personally visited by Rails-to-Trails Conservancy staff. Maps, photographs, and trail descriptions are as accurate as possible thanks to the work of the following contributors:

Annaly Galeas
Barbara Richey
Ben Carter
Bob Campbell
Carl Knoch
Cindy Dickerson
Elton Clark
Frederick Schaedtler
Gail Lipstein
Hardi Rosner
Jane Brookstein
Joseph Stark
Kartik Sribarra
Keith Laughlin
Lisa Diernisse
Mark Donofrio
Michelle Bosau
Milo Bateman
Pat Tomes
Patrick McKinney
Susan Weaver
Tim Rosner
Tom Sexton

Special thanks to Jeff Doppelt for his generous support of Rails-to-Trails Conservancy's guidebook program.

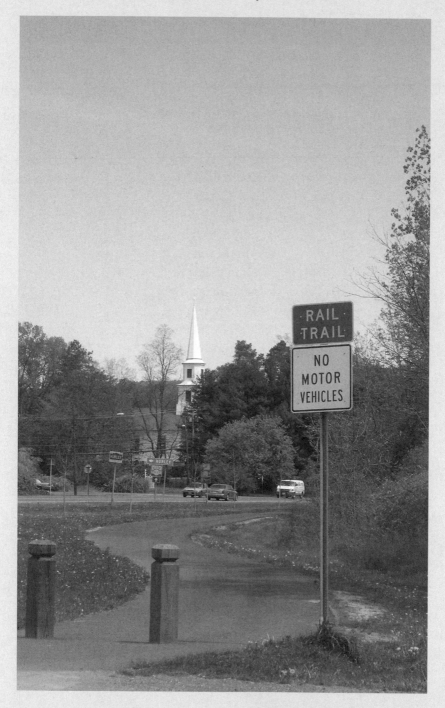

A trip on the D & H Canal Heritage Corridor include glimpses of the Catskill Mountains.

INDEX

A

Airplane Park (NY), 75, 76
Akron (NY), 61
Albany (NY), 100, 101
Allaire State Park (NJ), 17
Allamuchy Mountain State Park (NJ), 37
Allegheny (NY), 41
Allegheny National Forest (PA), 180
Allegheny Portage Railroad Trail (PA), 281
Allegheny River, 42, 155, 161, 173, 305, 307
Allegheny River Trail (PA), 154–156
Allegheny River Valley Trail (NY), 40–43
Allegheny State Park (NY), 117
Allegheny Valley Railroad, 155, 157, 161, 305
Allentown (PA), 251, 253, 277
Amenia (NY), 71–72
Amherst (NY), 61
Ancram (NY), 73
Anderson Creek (PA), 181
Andover (NJ), 37
Apollo (PA), 303
Appleseed, Johnny, 305
Arboretum Trail (PA), 157–159
Ardsley (NY), 125
Armstrong Trail (PA), 160–162
Ashfield (PA), 250
Atlantic & Great Western Railroad, 191
Atlantic City (NJ), 9, 10, 31
Atlantic County Bikeway (NJ), 8–10
Atlantic Highlands (NJ), 19
Auburn and Rochester Railroad, 46
Auburn Trail (NY), 44–47, 94, 96
Avon (NY), 69

B

Back Mountain Trail (PA), 163–165
Bald Eagle Mountain (PA), 263

Ballston (NY), 149
Ballston Lake (NY), 49
Ballston Veterans Bike Path (NY), 48–50
Bangor and Portland Railway, 293
Barton House (NY), 72
Bartram Trail (PA), 313
Bash Bish Falls (NY), 73
bathrooms map icon, 4
Beech Creek Railroad, 317
Bellefonte (PA), 167, 168
Bellefonte Central Rail Trail (PA), 166–168
Belmar Bridge (PA), 309
Berwick (PA), 329, 331
Bethlehem (PA), 275
Betzwood (PA), 312
Bicentennial Park (PA), 269, 271
Big Flats Trail (NY), 51–53
Black Creek Culvert (NY), 68
Black Creek (NY), 86
Black Diamond Trail (NY), 94
Blatnick Park (NY), 100
Bloomville (NY), 57, 59
Boalsburg (PA), 286
Bog Meadow Brook Nature Trail (NY), 54–56
book, how to use this, 3–6
Boston & Maine Railroad, 137
Brandon (PA), 155
Brewster (NY), 73, 103, 119, 120
Briarcliff Library (NY), 104
Bristol (PA), 169, 203, 251
Bristol Spurline Park (PA), 169–171
Brockway (PA), 179
Bronx, New York City, 107–108
Brooklyn Botanic Garden (NY), 104
Brookville (PA), 268
Butler (PA), 173–174
Butler-Freeport Community Trail (PA), 172–174, 348

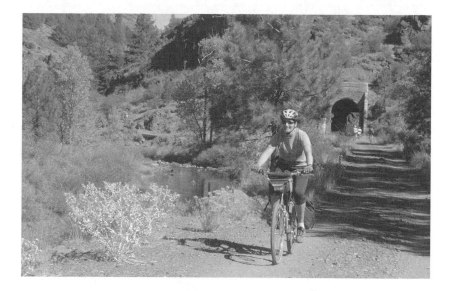

Become a member
of Rails-to-Trails Conservancy

As the nation's leader in helping communities transform unused railroad corridor into multiuse trails, Rails-to Trails Conservancy (RTC) depends on the support of its members and donors to create access to healthy outdoor experiences.

You can help support the future of rail-trails and enhance America's communities and countryside by becoming a member of Rails-to-Trails Conservancy today. Your donations will help support programs, projects and services that have helped put more than 19,000 rail-trail miles on the ground.

Every day, RTC provides vital technical assistance to communities throughout the country, advocates for trail-friendly policies at the local, state and national levels, promotes the benefits of rail-trails and defends rail-trail laws in the courts.

Join RTC in *"inspiring movement"* and receive the following benefits:

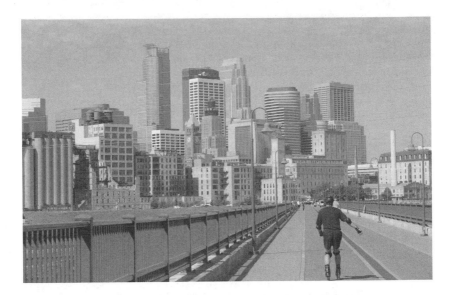

❶ New member welcome materials including *Destination Rail-Trails*, a sampler of some of the nation's finest trails.

❷ A **subscription** to RTC's quarterly magazine, *Rails to Trails*.

❸ **Dicounts** on publications, apparel and other merchandise including RTC's popular rail-trail guidebooks.

❹ The **satisfaction** of knowing that your dollars are helping to create a nationwide network of trails.

Membership benefits start at just $18, but additional contributions are gladly accepted.

Join online at **www.railstotrails.org**.

Join by mail by sending your contribution to Rails-to-Trails Conservancy, Attention: Membership, 2121 Ward Court, NW, 5th Floor, Washington, DC 20037.

Join by phone by calling 1-866-202-9788.

Contributions to Rails-to-Trails Conservancy are tax deductible to the full extent of the law.